Leading for **Health** and **Wellbeing**

You can find out more information on each of these titles and our other learning resources at www.sagepub.co.uk

Leading for Health and Wellbeing

Vicki Taylor

Series Editor:
Vicki Taylor

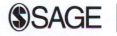

Los Angeles | London | New Delhi
Singapore | Washington DC

www.learningmatters.co.uk

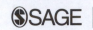

Los Angeles | London | New Delhi
Singapore | Washington DC

www.learningmatters.co.uk

Learning Matters
An imprint of Sage Publications Ltd
1 Oliver's Yard
55 City Road
London EC1Y 1SP

SAGE Publications Inc.
2455 Teller Road
Thousand Oaks, California 91320

Sage Publications India Pvt Ltd
B 1/I 1 Mohan Cooperative Industrial Area
Mathura Road
New Delhi 110 044

SAGE Publications Asia-Pacific Pte Ltd
3 Church Street
#10-04 Samsung Hub
Singapore 049483

Editor: Becky Taylor
Development editor: Ros Morley
Production controller: Chris Marke
Project management: Swales & Willis Ltd,
Exeter, Devon
Marketing manager: Tamara Navaratnam
Cover and text design: Code 5 Design Associates
Typeset by: Swales & Willis Ltd, Exeter, Devon
Printed by: TJ International Ltd, Padstow,
Cornwall

Library of Congress Central Number:
2011945609

British Library Cataloguing in Publication data

A catalogue record for this book is available
from the British Library

ISBN 978 0 85725 829 8
ISBN 978 0 85725 290 6 (pbk)

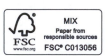

Contents

Foreword from the Series Editor

The publication of the Public Health Skills and Career Framework in April 2008 provided, for the first time, an overall framework for career development in public health in the United Kingdom. Prior to this, the focus had been primarily on the public health specialist workforce. The development of the framework itself was a truly collaborative enterprise involving a large number of organisations and stakeholder groups, and was designed to enable individuals at any stage of their career to identify a pathway for skills and career progression.

Within the framework, public health is divided into nine areas of work. There are four core areas that anyone working in public health must know about and within which they must have certain competences. There are five non-core or 'defined' areas, representing the contexts within which individuals principally work and develop.

Core areas	Non-core (defined) areas
Surveillance and assessment of the population's health and wellbeing	Health improvement
	Health protection
Assessing the evidence of effectiveness of interventions, programmes and services	Public health intelligence
Policy and strategy development and implementation	Academic public health
Leadership and collaborative working	Health and social care quality

This new series, 'Transforming Public Health Practice', has been developed as a direct response to development of the framework, and has a book dedicated to each of the four core areas of public health: *Measuring Health and Wellbeing, Assessing Evidence to Improve Population Health and Wellbeing, Policy and Strategy for Improving Health and Wellbeing,* and *Leading for Health and Wellbeing* are all featured.

The framework defines nine levels of competence and knowledge: level 1 will have little previous knowledge, skills or experience in public health, while those at level 9 will be setting strategic priorities and direction and providing leadership to improve population health and wellbeing. This series is aimed at those who want to develop their skills and knowledge in public health at levels 7–9 (which broadly equates to Master's level), although the series will be relevant to a wider group with the publication of the Public Health Practitioner standards and opening of the Public Health Practitioner Register. This will include those interested in acquiring or developing their public health competences and knowledge and, in particular, those who are seeking to demonstrate their public health skills and knowledge (and may be considering putting together a portfolio to demonstrate this at specialist or practitioner level).

This series will also be useful for anyone whose work involves improving people's health and wellbeing, or has a direct impact on the health and wellbeing of communities and populations – this encompasses a wide range of work areas, organisations and agencies.

Individual books in the series outline the key knowledge and skills in the core area and take further through case studies and scenarios how these competences can be used in practice. Activities and self-assessment tools are provided throughout the book, which will help the reader to hone their critical thinking and reflection skills.

Chapters in each of the books follow a standard format. At the beginning a box highlights links to relevant competences. This sets the scene and enables the reader to see exactly what will be covered. This is extended by a chapter overview, which sets out the key topics and what the reader should expect to have learnt by the end of the chapter.

There is usually at least one case study in each chapter, which considers public health skills and knowledge in practice. Activities such as practical tasks with learning points, critical thinking and reflective practice are included. Each activity is followed by a brief commentary on the issues raised. At the end of each chapter, a summary provides a reminder of what has been covered.

All the chapters are evidence-based in that they set out the theory or evidence that underpins practice. In most chapters, one or more 'What's the evidence?' boxes provide further information. A list of additional readings is set out under the 'Going further' section, with all references collated at the end of the book.

In summary, this series will provide invaluable support to anyone studying or practising in the field of public health, in a range of different settings.

Vicki Taylor
Independent Public Health Consultant and Director,
The Roundhouse Consultancy, MK Ltd
Associate Lecturer, The Open University
Previously Senior Lecturer, London Southbank University,
Senior Lecturer, Kings College, London

Author Information

John Harvey is a director of a limited company providing public health consultancy. He trained as a public health consultant after working for nine years in Yemen, doing mainly maternal and child health programmes. He has experience as a director of public health in three different settings – Newcastle, Jersey, and the London Borough of Havering – where he was a visiting professor of public health at London South Bank University. He is an honorary Fellow of the Royal College of Paediatrics and Child Health, and the co-chair of the Child Public Health Interest Group for the Faculty of Public Health.

Vivien Martin's current post is at the University of Brighton Business School. Her background is in adult learning, training and development: she was an Area Principal in Adult Education, a Principal Lecturer in Management Development in the University of Brighton, and became Director of Management Education in the South Thames NHS Region through the 1990s. She joined the Open University to lead a project with the Department of Health to revise open learning materials for management development, and then moved into the NHS Leadership Centre.

Susie Sykes is a senior lecturer at London South Bank University, where she teaches on the MSc programme in Public Health and Health Promotion. With a background in health promotion and public health, Susie has experience of working in both the voluntary and public sectors. Her areas of particular interest are community development, policymaking and health literacy. She is currently research active on her PhD, exploring the concept of critical health literacy.

Vicki Taylor has worked in public health since 1985 in a range of different roles at local, regional and national levels, and is now Director of the Roundhouse Consultancy MK Ltd. She has a strong interest in public health development and, in particular, the development of public health leadership and management. She has substantive experience of public health and public health practitioner development in a number of geographical areas, spanning a period of more than 25 years. Vicki is an assessor for the UK Public Health Register and has experience of assessing public health portfolios at consultant and practitioner level. Currently she is providing Learning Sets and support for the West Midlands Public Health Practitioner's Pilot Assessment Scheme and the Kent and Medway Public Health Practitioner's Pilot Assessment Scheme, and will be providing Learning Sets for a new scheme in Surrey and Sussex. Vicki was the project manager for the NHS South Central public health practitioner development scheme from March 2007 until November 2009. In these roles Vicki has influenced the development of public health practitioner schemes.

Rhonda Ware is a registered nurse who has worked at a senior level in the commercial, charity, local authority and health sectors, including private and the NHS. Rhonda was a senior manager in public health, having previous expertise in children's health and education, learning disabilities and care of the elderly. She is now Co-Director of Tiger Health Limited, which offers consultancy in healthcare and public health. Rhonda has a particular interest in leadership and change management, governance and quality improvement.

Steve Whiteman is the Deputy Director of Public Health for Greenwich, and has worked in the NHS in south-east London for 17 years. Throughout this time he has worked closely with Greenwich

Council and other strategic partners to develop and implement programmes of cross-agency work to improve health and wellbeing in the borough. He has been a principal author of the borough's health and wellbeing strategy, and is the chair of a number of strategic partnership groups, such as the Greenwich Men's Health Forum and the Learning Disability Health Partnership Group. He has held management and leadership roles for public health since 1997. Building sustainable cross-agency partnerships and developing joint strategies to address complex public health challenges has always been central to his approach.

Introduction
Vicki Taylor

'Making change actually happen takes leadership.'
Lord Darzi, 2008, High Quality of Care for All,
NHS Next Stage Review Final Report

Public health and health promotion are essentially about leadership and achieving change, changes that will improve health. Leadership to improve public health is a complex process requiring leadership across organisations and an ability to engage with a wide range of people and organisations.

Leadership for health and health improvement is complex on a number of levels. The need to work with multiple stakeholders, and to lead effectively across organisations in order to promote health requires an increasing understanding of complexity and leadership skills. Over the last decade there has been a growing awareness of the importance of leadership in promoting health.

The development of a national strategy for Public Health leadership in the UK demonstrates recognition of the importance of leadership skills in achieving public health outcomes. This strategy (for public health leadership) was based on the development of a 'network of individuals across the NHS and partner organisations, skilled in the areas of health improvement'.

Building on the core competences for public health, this book focuses on leadership and collaborative working to improve health and wellbeing and adds to the existing literature. Key themes identified within this book relate to the paucity of leadership theory within the health promotion and public health literature and the necessity to draw on wider leadership and management theory. Writing about leadership development in 1997, Catford notes that, *there is an absolute paucity of research on what makes good public health leaders and how leadership can be strengthened* (*Catford*, 1997, p2). Hannaway et al. (2009, p206) note the limited literature on public health leadership and leadership development.

Activities are included throughout the book to encourage the reader to stop, to reflect on and to critically examine their own leadership practice.

Is this book for me?

This book is one of a series of four books aimed at addressing the core standards for public health practice as set out in the UK Public Health Skills and Career Framework (2004). It covers the second core area in the Public Health Skills and Career Framework: 'Leadership and collaborative working to improve population health and wellbeing'.

Bringing together key leadership and theory, models and frameworks, this book provides a practical resource that can be applied to public health and health promotion practice. It aims to make accessible from the vast leadership and management literature some key concepts that may have relevance to public health leadership. Through the use of case studies and activities, this book seeks to support the achievement of health improvement and health promotion goals. It is hoped that approach taken gives the reader an opportunity to consider ways of contributing to leadership for health improvement.

The primary aim of the authors is to create a practical resource to support anyone preparing a portfolio for submission for registration as a defined specialist (at level 8), or registration as a public health practitioner (at level 5) and for those who are interested in the standards for leadership for health.

How the book works

This book is organised into nine chapters. A consideration of 'Leadership' and theory about leadership is at the heart of Chapters 1 and 2. In Chapter 1 the focus is on more traditional models of leadership. Chapter 2 introduces leadership as a dynamic social process and proposes that it might offer a greater understanding of public health leadership. Chapter 3 seeks to develop a wider understanding of organisations and the different organisational stuctures and cultures that can exist. It is suggested that an understanding of organisations and how they work helps public health professionals to be more effective participants in, and leaders of, organisations. In Chapter 4 the emphasis shifts to the challenge of leading partnerships and working across organisational boundaries effectively. Leadership skills such as negotiation, persuasion and influencing and the nature of power are considered in Chapter 5. The importance of understanding one's self and the communication process in order to increase effectiveness in promoting and securing health improvement are also emphasised.

Chapter 6 considers what the term leadership means when working in a community context. A range of different models for working in and with communities to improve health and wellbeing are presented. Identifying the potential challenges that may exist in this kind of work and enabling the reader to identify strategies for overcoming these challenges are integral to the activities in this chapter.

Chapter 7 utilises a health improvement leadership framework as a template for understanding the skills needed to lead public health at a local level. The arguments are structured around three dimensions: professional, political and people.

The final two chapters are intended to help the reader to develop their thinking about managing projects and leading and managing change to improve health. In both chapters theory is used to generate practical frameworks and models that can assist the reader to implement change and to manage public health projects.

How to use this book

You may be using this book to help prepare a portfolio for registration as a defined specialist (at level 8), registration as a public health practitioner (at level 5) or you may be using this book as part of your studies. Once you are clear about the focus or standard you wish to consider, whether (for example) it is knowledge of various leadership styles, look at the table below which gives you a quick guide to the chapter titles and the standards (UK Public Health Skills and Career Framework (PHSCF), National Occupational Standards (NOS) and Public Health Practitioner Standards (PHPS)) covered within the chapter. A chapter overview, at the beginning of each chapter, augments this information and sets you in the right direction.

Chapters, UK Public Health Skills and Career Framework (PHSCF), National Occupational Standards (NOS) and Public Health Practitioner Standards (PHPS)

Chapter	PHSCF (knowledge and skills)	NOS	PHPS
1 Leadership – what is it?	5(2), 5(d), 5(e), 6(a), 7(b), 8(1), 8(a), 8(f)	(M&L_B5), (M&L_B6), (PHP45), (PHS20), (M&L_B7)	Standard 11 a), b), c) i, ii, iii
2 Leadership as a social process	5(2), 5(d), 5(e), 6(a), 7(b), 8(1), 8(2), 8(a), 8(f)	(M&L_B5), (M&L_B6), (PHP45), (PHS09), (M&L_B7)	Standard 11 a), b), c) i, ii, iii
3 Working in and with organisations	5(1), 5(3), 5(5), 5(j), 6(5), 7(2), 8(1), 8(2), 8(b), 8(c)	(M&L_B2), (M&L_D2), (PHS10), (M&L_B9)	Standard 11 b), c), i, ii, iii
4 Leading strategic partnerships	5(a), 6(b), 6(2), 7(2), 7(7), 7(a), 8(6), 8(c), 8(d)	(SfJ_AD2), (M&L_B2), (M&L_D2), (PHS09)	Standard 9, Standard 11 a), b), c), i, ii, iii
5 Skills for leading	5(2), 5(3), 5(6) 5(b), 6(f), 7(2), 7(5), 7(e), 7(f), 8(3)	(M&L_B5), (M&L_B6), (SfJ AD1), (PHP47), (CJ_F408), (PHS11)	Standard 11 a), b), Standard 12
6 Leading communities collaboratively	5(1), 6(1), 6(2), 6(6), 6(a), 6(b), 7(2), 7(3), 7(2), 7(7), 7(a), 8(1), 8(6), 8(7), 8(a)	(M&L_B5), (M&L_B6), (SfJ AD1), (PHP45)	Standard 11 c), i
7 Leading at a local level	5(5), 6(5), 6(d), 7(1), 7(3), 7(8), 7(9), 7(h), 8(1), 8(h)	(M&L_B5), (M&L_B6), (PHP45), (PHS09), (M&L_B7)	Standard 11 a), b), c), i, ii, iii Standard 12
8 Leading and managing projects	5(3), 6(3), 6(c), 7(1), 7(3)	(M&L_F1), (M&L_F2)	Standard 10 d)
9 Leading and managing change	5(4), 5(g), 6(4), 6(g), 6(h), 7(4), 7(g), 8(5), 8(g)	(M&L_C4), (M&L_C5), (M&L_C6)	Standard 10 d)
These competences are covered in the book as whole:	5(f), 5(j)		

M&L=Management & Leadership; PHP = public health practice; PHS = public health specialists; SfJ = Skills for Justice Common; CJ = Community Justice

chapter 1

Leadership: What Is It?

Vicki Taylor

Meeting the Public Health Competences

This chapter will help you to evidence the following competences for public health (Public Health Skills and Career Framework):

- Level 5(2) Lead on discrete areas of work;
- Level 5(d) Knowledge of various leadership styles;
- Level 5(e) Knowledge of the difference between management and leadership;
- Level 5(h) Understanding of your interaction with and impact on others;
- Level 6(a) Knowledge of the models and principles of leadership and their application;
- Level 7(b) Understanding of the models and principles of leadership and their potential use in improving population health and wellbeing;
- Level 8(1) Lead on improving population health and wellbeing within and/or across organisations;
- Level 8(a) Understanding of the models and principles of leadership and their potential use in improving and protecting health and wellbeing and in motivating colleagues and partners;
- Level 8(f) Understanding of basic management models and theories associated with motivation and leadership.

This chapter will also assist you in demonstrating the following National Occupational Standards for public health:

- Provide leadership for your team (M&L_B5);
- Provide leadership in your area of responsibility (M&L_B6);
- Lead others in improving health and wellbeing (PHP45);
- Lead teams and individuals to improve health and wellbeing (PHS20);
- Provide leadership for your organisation (M&L_B7).

In addition, this chapter will be useful in demonstrating Standard 11 of the Public Health Practitioner Standards:

Standard 11. Work collaboratively with people from teams and agencies other than one's own to improve health and wellbeing outcomes – demonstrating:

a. awareness of personal impact on others;
b. constructive relationships with a range of people who contribute to population health and wellbeing;
c. awareness of:

i. the principles of effective partnership working;

ii. the ways in which organisations, teams and individuals work together to improve health and wellbeing outcomes;

iii. the different forms that teams might take.

Overview

This chapter will help you to consider what leadership means and the implications for leading public health and health improvement. It will also help you to develop your thinking about the nature of leadership and how it differs from management. In this chapter we will consider the relationship between leadership and management and review some of the more traditional approaches to leadership, from trait and 'style' theories of leadership to approaches that view leadership as situational or dependent upon the situation in which leaders find themselves. Finally, we will consider some key challenges in leading public health programmes, and look at the implications for public health leadership.

The activities in this chapter will focus on:

• clarifying the differences between leadership and management;
• understanding why there is no one best way to lead;
• exploring a range of models and definitions of leadership;
• appreciating the strengths and weaknesses of different approaches to leadership and their potential use in improving population health and wellbeing.

This chapter uses theory, tools and case studies to explore leadership and management.

After reading this chapter you will be able to:

• articulate the difference between leadership and management;
• identify a range of models and definitions of leadership;
• appreciate the strengths and weaknesses of different approaches to leadership;
• identify key challenges for public health leadership.

The relationship between leadership and management

Leadership is a topic that captures the public imagination and is regularly talked about: there are countless books, articles and publications about leadership, but no common agreement on what it is. It seems to be one of those concepts that we talk about, but find difficult to describe. Exploring the relationship between leadership and management might help to provide a clearer understanding of leadership.

Leadership and management are often used interchangeably, but to what extent are they the same thing? The answer you give to this question depends very much on your view of both management and leadership. There are a range of views about the differences and similarities between management and leadership.

ACTIVITY 1.1

Spend a few minutes thinking about your own experience of management and leadership, then consider the following questions.

What is management? What is leadership?

What do you see as the key tasks of a manager and a leader?

Do good managers make good leaders?

Do good leaders make good managers?

Comment

Martin *et al.* (2010) suggest that there are three frequently discussed ways of viewing the relationship between leadership and management. The first view sees management and leadership as the same thing (view 1 in Figure 1.1 below). This view is not as widely supported as it once was, and most people now make a distinction between leadership and management, arguing that these are not interchangeable. The second view sees management as a component of leadership (view 2), and the third view sees leadership as a subset of management (view 3). In his consideration of the roles that managers undertake, Mintzberg (1973) appears to share this third view, where he describes leadership as one of ten sub-roles of management rather than as a category in its own right.

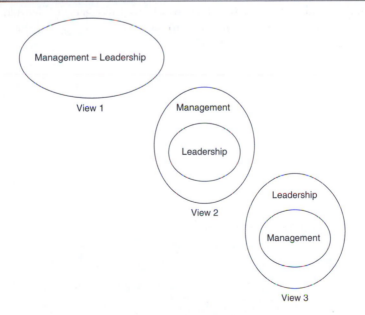

Figure 1.1 The relationship between leadership and management

Looking at the literature on leadership in more detail, two other ways of viewing the relationship between leadership and management emerge. One perspective is to view the two concepts as distinct from one another, and the other suggests that there is some overlap (as represented in Figure 1.2).

Whichever of these views of leadership and management you hold, currently there is general agreement that leading and managing are different enterprises. Bennis and Nanus (1985) state that there is a profound difference between management and leadership, and both are important. For Bennis and Nanus, to manage means to bring about, accomplish, have charge of or responsibility for conduct. Leading is influencing, guiding in a direction, course, action or opinion: *Managers are people who do things right* while *leaders are people who do the right thing* (1985, p221). Covey shares this view, stating that *Management focuses on speed and methods – doing things right. Leadership focuses on direction and purpose – doing the right things* (1989, p101).

Zaleznik (1977) argues that management and leadership are distinct activities requiring different skills and capabilities. He sees managers and leaders as being fundamentally different types of people who operate and think in very different ways. Leaders, he says, seek change and in doing so, do not need managerial structures or a sense of closure; they can tolerate or even create chaos. Managers seek order and control, and try to achieve closure of problems as quickly as possible. Leadership is concerned with vision, a sense of direction and the commitment of others, while management is the process of organising people and resources to achieve goals.

Kotter (1990) distinguishes between managers as being concerned with *transactions* and leaders as being concerned with *transformation*. Kotter argues that both managers and leaders need to determine what needs to be done, develop the capacity to do it and ensure that it is done. However, there is a clear distinction between the way that managers and leaders deal with these functions. Managers decide what needs to be done through a process of planning, while leaders focus on setting the

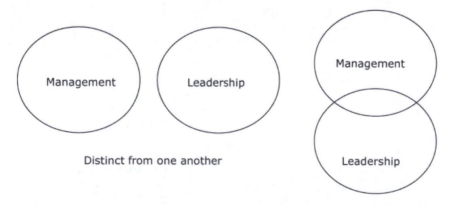

Figure 1.2 The relationship between leadership and management – additional perspectives

direction and creating the vision. In developing the capacity to do it, managers focus on organising and staffing, whereas leaders focus on aligning people, communicating the vision and enabling others to make the vision a reality. In ensuring that the task is done managers solve problems and control, whereas leaders are concerned with motivating and inspiring others and producing change. Northouse (1997) notes that leadership and management are similar in some ways, but that they are also quite different. For example, they both involve influence and require working with people, but they are different from one another, with management producing order and consistency, and leadership producing change and movement.

Table 1.1 provides a summary of the differences between management and leadership identified by Kotter (1990) and Northouse (1997). Look back at your response to Activity 1.1 and see whether you identified any of these differences.

Table 1.1 Differences between management and leadership

Management	*Leadership*
Produces order, consistency and predictability	Produces positive and sometimes dramatic change and movement
Planning, budgeting	Vision-building, strategising
Organising, staffing	Aligning people, communicating
Controlling, problem-solving, corrective action	Motivating, inspiring, empowering and energising

Source: Adapted from Northouse (1997) and Kotter (1990)

In summary, contemporary ideas about leadership and management share a consensus that leading and managing are different, but whether they are distinct is less clear. As mentioned previously, management roles involve managers planning, organising and controlling work, while leaders are usually concerned with change and creating vision. Although leaders do not have to be managers, many managers are often required to display leadership capability.

Martin *et al.* (2010, p30) suggest that a useful way of seeing the relationship between managers and leaders is to think of these roles as being added to other roles. For example, we can think of teachers, nurses, epidemiologists, health visitors, public health analysts, environmental health officers, health promotion and social marketing taking on an additional role as a manager. Each of these also might take the lead on discrete areas of work, or be members of different teams in which they take on different roles based on expertise, experience and skills.

What is leadership?

Public health professionals are regularly required to lead initiatives to improve health at a local level. So what, then, is leadership? In this section we will explore the nature of leadership, but first let's focus on someone you consider to be a leader.

ACTIVITY 1.2

If you were asked to describe a leader you admire, who would you think of and why?

What makes you see them as a leader? Who they are? What they have achieved? Is it where they operate? How they get things done?

Comment

The literature on leadership is extensive, and there are many theoretical approaches that aim to make sense of leadership. Some of these theories focus on the personal qualities and characteristics that a leader has, and are often referred to as trait theories. Another group of theories define leadership by the way in which the leader does the job, how they exercise the different functions of leadership. Table 1.2 below illustrates these approaches to leadership.

Look back at your response to Activity 1.2 and see whether you defined leadership in terms of personal characteristics, style or functions.

Table 1.2 Common approaches to leadership

Personal characteristics	A focus on the inherent characteristics of a leader – Trait theory
Leadership style	A focus on the behaviour of a leader, the way in which they lead – Leadership behaviour, leadership style
Functions of leadership	How the functions of leadership are carried out

In the next section, a summary of some of the more traditional approaches to leadership (trait, style, situational and contingency theories) is presented. We begin by looking at theories that focus on the characteristics of successful leaders, then move on to examine theories that are concerned with how leaders behave. Next, we look at situational and contingency theories of leadership. These emphasise that different situations require different types of leadership, and that effective leadership is where a leader chooses an appropriate leadership style to suit the context or situation in which they are leading. All of these theories of leadership have a focus on the leaders and an in-built assumption of a hierarchical relationship between leaders and followers.

As you encounter each of these different approaches to leadership you might like to critically review their strengths and weaknesses, and consider the extent to which they have relevance for public health leadership.

Trait theories of leadership

Theories that are concerned with leaders' characteristics or qualities are referred to as 'trait theories', since much of the early research concentrated on the innate qualities that leaders were seen to possess. The assumption underlying these theories is that what makes someone an effective leader is their personality and personal qualities. Leaders are people who display particular characteristics or traits (Bass, 1990; Gardner, 1990; Grint, 1997; McKimm and Philips, 2009). Leaders were often described as charismatic and as possessing leadership qualities (Kirkpatrick and Locke, 1991; Mullins, 2002; Fulop *et al.*, 2004). One of the criticisms of this view of leadership is the implication that leaders need to be selected, rather than developed.

ACTIVITY 1.3

Think about a public health leader that you know well. What are the key characteristics that you would expect to see in this person?

Look at the job description for a public health leader. What characteristics, if any, are identified?

What does this tell you about leadership?

What does this tell you about public health leadership?

Numerous studies have identified different traits, but only a few of these are common to different studies. There is some consensus that intelligence, initiative, self-confidence, integrity, an orientation towards achievement and interpersonal skills are important, although there is no universal agreement on the relative importance of these factors. Dissatisfaction with this approach began to surface as researchers identified traits found in leaders that appeared to be inconsistent, contradictory or correlating little with one another (Mullins, 2002). Coupled with the growing view that it is the way that a leader behaves rather than their characteristics that makes them effective leaders, these criticisms have led to attempts to identify the most effective way for leaders to behave.

Style or behavioural theories of leadership

Researchers began to search for those behaviours that characterised effective leaders. The research focus shifted from identifying characteristics to a focus on what leaders do. Different patterns of behaviour were grouped together and labelled as 'styles'. Style theories of leadership focus on the style that leaders adopt, and suggest that certain styles are more effective than others in getting followers to work hard or achieve the desired performance.

What's the evidence?

Lewin, Lippitt and white (1939) research looked at different styles of leadership in a boy's club. They studied three different styles:

1. *autocratic* – where the leader decides what will be done and how;
2. *democratic* – in which decisions are made after discussion;
3. *laissez-faire* – where team members work on their own and the leader keeps their participation to a minimum.

In these different situations the team was most productive under an autocratic leader. However, under this style the leader needed to be present, or the work stopped. A democratic style was the most popular and the most consistent in both quality and performance. The laissez-faire style rated poorly both in terms of quality and productivity; however, this style can be effective where team members are clear about their objectives, roles and the task that they are undertaking.

One of the most influential style leadership frameworks was developed by Blake and Mouton (1978), and later refined by Blake and McCanse (1991). They synthesised the work of a number of researchers to develop their leadership styles grid. This grid classifies leadership styles according to two dimensions: production and people. The extent to which a leader demonstrates *behaviour* relating to production (concern for the task to be achieved or getting the job done) and concern for people, is plotted on two axes on a scale from low to high (1–9). Blake and Mouton proposed that, irrespective of context, the most effective leaders show a high concern for both tasks and people, as represented by position (9.9) on the grid.

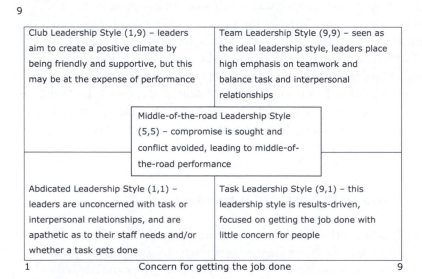

Figure 1.3 Leadership styles

Source: Adapted from Blake and Mouton (1978)

ACTIVITY 1.4

Looking at your own organisation, is there a particular leadership style or is there a variety of styles?

With what leadership style do you most strongly identify? Are you more concerned for people or production?

Can you identify situations where each of these leadership styles might be appropriate?

How might these be relevant for public health?

Comment

You may have identified that you use a mixture of styles depending on the situation, even though you may have a preference for one. In practice, most leaders' concern for getting the job done and concern for people varies considerably from one situation or context to another.

Martin (2003) gives the following description and examples for each of Blake and Mouton's leadership style.

Position (1,9) 'Social Club Leader'

Lack of conflict and general wellbeing are considered more important than achieving.

This is often a popular style of management with staff and service users in situations where achieving tasks is less critical: for example, in a long-term care situation.

Position (9,1) 'Task Leader'

People are expected to perform as machines whose only purpose is to complete the task. The leader's responsibility is to plan, supervise and control the work.

In emergencies this style is appropriate: for example, in an ambulance service there may be times when quick and efficient action with little or no discussion is essential.

Position (1,1) 'Abdicated Leader'

Little effort is expended on either people or the task, leaving an absence of leadership and little motivation for people to work. A lack of decision-making encourages conflict or indifference at work.

This situation might be found if there has been no lead for some time and people feel unable to take the lead.

Position (9,9) 'Team Leader'

This is often considered the ideal style to adopt, with high concern for both people and the task. This position should represent commitment to a common purpose and achievement through involvement and participation.

Position (5,5) 'Maintenance Leader'

There is some attempt to achieve the task, but with only moderate effort from the workforce. This might happen when everyone is tired after a major effort and represents maintenance rather than progression. This may be a politically expedient position to adopt from time to time, but the emphasis is on maintaining balance rather than making any change or progress.

Source: Adapted from Martin (2003)

One of the main criticisms of style or behavioural theories of leadership has been that they tend to ignore the importance of the context in which leadership takes place. This led to the development of theories of leadership that take into account the situations in which leaders lead. The awareness that different contexts and different situations require different approaches to leadership have led to views of leadership that are more context-specific, often referred to as situational and contingency theories of leadership.

Situational and contingency leadership theories

Situational theories

Situational theories focus on leadership *in situations* (Northouse, 1997, p55). This view of leadership is based on the notion that different situations require different types of leadership. Effective leaders are those who adopt their style to best fit the situation. A key situational variable is the developmental level of followers (Hersey and Blanchard, 1988[1969]). 'Developmental level' refers to the degree to which followers have the competence and commitment to perform a given task. Hersey and Blanchard proposed four leadership styles – telling, selling, participating and delegating – that matched followers' developmental level. These different styles were based on the degree of supportive and directive behaviours that the leader needed to influence followers.

Leaders need to diagnose the follower's maturity level in relation to the particular task and adapt their leadership style to match this (Northouse, 2001, pp58–9). From this perspective, leaders need to be flexible in their leadership behaviour and adapt their style to suit their followers and their unique situations. The effective leader is someone who ensures that the leadership style that they adopt fits the situation that they face (summarised in Table 1.3).

The four leadership styles

Telling *(high task/low relationship behaviour)*

This style or approach is characterised by providing direction to subordinates and by giving considerable attention to defining roles and goals. The style is recommended for dealing with new staff, where the work is menial or repetitive, or where things have to be completed within a short time span. Subordinates are viewed as being unable or unwilling to perform independently.

Selling *(high task/high relationship behaviour)*

In this approach most of the direction is provided by the leader; however, there is an attempt to encourage people to take on the task. This is used when people are willing and motivated, but lack the required maturity or ability.

Participating *(high relationship/low task behaviour)*

Decision-making is shared between leaders and followers, with the leader facilitating the process. It involves high support and low direction, and is used when people are able but insecure.

Delegating *(low relationship/low task behaviour)*

The leader identifies the problem or issue and responsibility is given to followers. Followers have a high degree of competence and confidence, and are motivated to achieve.

Table 1.3 Summary of situational leadership

	Leadership style	*Leader subordinate/follower*
Telling	Provides clear instruction and direction	Low follower readiness level, unable, unwilling or insecure
Selling	Encourages two-way communication, builds confidence and motivation but retains control	Moderate follower readiness level, unable but willing or confident
Participating	Shares decision-making with followers	Moderate follower readiness level, able but insecure
Delegating	Passes responsibility to followers	High follower readiness level, able, willing or confident

Source: Adapted from Hersey and Blanchard (1988)

Contingency theories

These are based on the belief that there is no single style of leadership appropriate to all situations. They argue that effective leadership is dependent on the context in which a leader is leading. There is a focus on identifying the contextual variables that best predict the most appropriate leadership style to fit the particular leadership situation. One of the first contingency theories developed was the leadership continuum model by Tannenbaum and Schmidt (1958, 1973), who proposed that leaders adapt their style to suit the situation, choosing from a continuum of leadership styles that range from autocratic (boss-centred) to democratic (subordinate-centred). The more democratic the leadership style, the greater the amount of follower participation, involvement and responsibility. Four main styles of leadership were identified: *tells, sells, consults* and *joins*, and seven positions along the continuum were identified.

Tannenbaum and Schmidt Leadership Continuum Model: '7 Positions'

1. The leader makes the decision and announces it (tells).
2. The leader makes the decision and sells it (sells).
3. The leader presents the decision and invites questions (discusses).
4. The leader presents a provisional decision and invites discussion before making the decision (negotiates).
5. The leader presents the problem, gets suggestions and then makes the decision (consults).
6. The leader explains the problem, defines the boundaries and delegates the decision to the team (delegates).
7. The leader allows the team to identify the problem and determine boundaries and make the decision (participates or collaborates).

Source: Adapted from Tannenbaum and Schmidt (1973), van Maurick (2001, pp9–11) and Martin (2003)

The steps in this continuum are presented as alternatives for the leader to choose from (Buchanan and Huzyznski, 2004) with the appropriate style contingent on three variables:

- *forces in the leader* – their personality and preferred style, value systems and confidence in subordinates;

- *forces in the subordinates* – the needs, attitudes and skills of the subordinates, team members or colleagues, degree of tolerance for ambiguity, readiness to assume responsibility for decision-making;

- *forces in the context* – the organisation, its values and prejudices, group effectiveness, nature of the problem, pressure of time.

ACTIVITY 1.5

Can you identify situations in which you would use these different leadership styles? How might this be applicable to leading public health and health improvement?

Comment

It is important to note that all of these styles are considered to be potentially useful ones to adopt, depending on the circumstances. No one style is better than another – just more, or less, appropriate to the situation. The key challenge for leadership for public health and health improvement is to identify the most appropriate style of leadership for the situation.

Emotional intelligence as a basis for enhancing leadership performance

Looking at how leaders lead and what makes the difference between average performance and outstanding performance, Goleman (1998, 2000; Goleman *et al.*, 2001, 2002) found that emotional intelligence (defined as *the capacity for recognising our own feelings and those of others, for motivating ourselves, for managing emotions well in ourselves and in our relationships*, Goleman, 1998, p317) was the biggest differentiator. Goleman describes four key competencies that underpin and enhance leadership performance.

1. *Self-awareness* – this is at the heart of the model and underpins the other quadrants. This is our ability to understand ourselves, our emotions, drives, strengths and weaknesses.

2. *Self-management* – this is about exercising self-control, but also about harnessing our drives to motivate ourselves. Lack of self-control has been found to be the main factor that prevents high-potential leaders from achieving their full potential.

3. *Social awareness* – this is about having empathy with others at both the individual and group levels.

4. *Relationship management* – the characteristics in this quadrant are most directly related to having a positive impact on others. Relationship management requires the foundation of the other quadrants.

(*Source*: Hay ECI accreditation training)

In this model, self-awareness underpins self-management and social awareness, and these in turn underpin relationship management. Based on research conducted by Hay/McBer in which 3,871 executives were sampled randomly from a global database of 20,000, Goleman (2000) subsequently identified six leadership styles, each deriving from different components of emotional intelligence. These six leadership styles have been developed since and are summarised in Table 1.4 (Goleman *et al.*, 2003). The first four, *Visionary, Coaching, Affiliative, Democratic*, all emphasise listening and are referred to as 'resonance builders', unlike the 'dissonance' styles *Pacesetting* and *Commanding*, which do not have this emphasis.

Table 1.4 Leadership styles identified by Goleman *et al.* (2003)

Leadership style	Key features	Use	Impact on performance
Resonance builders			
Visionary	Inspires people, has a focus on long-term goals Listens to the values held by individuals Explains overall goals in a way that gains support	Transformational change Provides clear direction	Very strong positive impact
Coaching	Involves delegating, listening to employees Establishes personal rapport and trust, and helps others work out for themselves the best ways of working	Builds individual capabilities	Highly positive impact
Affiliative	Listens to discover emotional needs and to strives to fulfil these in the workplace Leader creates harmony and builds relationships	Resolves conflict Promotes trust Creates team bond Best used for getting though stressful situations	Can focus too much on emotional climate and not enough on the work itself Positive impact
Democratic	Values inputs and commitment via participation	Gets commitment through whole-team engagement Best used to gain buy-in or when simple inputs are needed	Positive impact
Dissonant styles			
Pacesetting	High standards for performance are set They tend to be low on guidance, expecting people to know what to do	Motivates around tasks Results-driven People get exhausted and burn out Done badly, it lacks emotional intelligence, especially self-management	Can have a negative impact if used poorly
Commanding	Issues instructions without asking for input on what is to be done or how	Can be useful in times of crisis and overcoming inertia Useful to manage poor performance Erodes motivation and commitment	Negative impact

The research also suggests that leaders with the best results do not rely on one style alone. Rather, they use them selectively in different measure and combination, depending on the circumstances in which they find themselves. Goleman concludes that those leaders who can use four or more styles effectively, in particular the *Visionary*, *Coaching*, *Affiliative* and *Democratic* styles, tend to foster a more productive work climate and thus achieve the best results (Goleman, 2000). The *Commanding* and *Pacesetting* styles are the least effective overall, but are useful in some situations. For example, *Pacesetting* can be useful for setting performance standards, and *Commanding* can be effective in a crisis situation.

ACTIVITY 1.6

How might developing greater insight into your own emotional intelligence enable you to be more effective in delivering public health and health improvement?

To what extent are you aware of your impact on others?

Which of the leadership styles suggested by Goleman do you use, and in what situations?

Comment

You may have identified that you use a mixture of styles depending on the situation, even though you may have a preference for one. You also may have identified the importance of having a greater awareness and understanding of yourself and others as a key requirement for effective delivery of public health work. In his consideration of leadership, Friedman suggests that one of the key things that public health leaders can do is to *acknowledge and work with their own emotions* (2011, p155) and those of others.

Fiedler (1967) supported the idea that the appropriate leadership style depends on the situation, although he did not subscribe to the view that leaders could easily change their leadership style to suit the situation. Instead, he proposed that leaders tend to be task-oriented or relationship-oriented, and that these different leadership styles are suited to different situations depending on the 'favourableness' of the situation. Fiedler identified three elements that collectively determine whether the situation is favourable to the leader:

1. whether the leader is liked and trusted by those being led (leader–member relations);

2. whether the task is clearly defined and clearly structured (task structure);

3. the power that the leader has and their capacity to exercise authority through reward or punishment (leader's position power).

Fiedler found that in the most favourable situations, all three of these elements are strong. Task-oriented managers tend to do better in situations that have good leader–member relationships, structured tasks and either weak or strong position power. They do well when the task is unstructured but position power is strong. They also do well at the other end of the spectrum, when leader–member relations are moderate to poor and the task unstructured. Relationship-oriented managers do better in all other situations and are most effective in moderately favourable situations (Linstead *et al.*, 2004).

From this perspective, understanding leaders' performance requires an understanding of the situations in which they lead and how favourable the situation is. Fiedler maintained that changing the favourableness of the situation by increasing the leader's authority or improving the structure of the task was the key to increasing leadership effectiveness.

ACTIVITY 1.7

Review the last section on situational and contingency theories of leadership. How do they differ from one another?

In what ways are they similar?

What are their relative strengths and weaknesses?

How might they be relevant for public health leadership?

Make a list of key points for your own learning. What are the implications for your own practice? How might you apply this in practice?

Comment

For many, situational and contingency theories are synonymous with one another, which is why you may have found the last activity difficult. Others see the two as distinct from one another. Table 1.5 is an attempt to compare the two approaches.

Table 1.5 Situational and contingency theories of leadership compared

Situational	Contingency
Sees leadership as being specific to the situation in which it is being undertaken.	Based on belief that there is no single style of leadership appropriate to all situations.
Concentrates on the importance of the situation and context in which leadership takes place.	Focus on identifying particular situational variables related to the environment which might determine the most appropriate style of leadership to fit the situation or circumstances.
Focus on leaders choosing the best approach based on situational variables.	

Different styles of leadership may be more appropriate for the situation and at different levels within the same organisation.

Effective leadership depends on leadership style, followers' qualities, the leadership situation and context.

Both contingency and situational theories take the view that the effectiveness of a leader's style is dependent on the situation or context in which leadership takes place. Both embrace a sharp distinction between leaders and followers and tend to view leadership as a hierarchical relationship.

Neither provides insight into how leadership is exercised when there is no formal hierarchy. They do not consider the possibility that people other than the leader might have a leadership role. The strategic dimensions of leadership, such as developing vision and direction, are not considered.

ACTIVITY 1.8

What do you see as the most important challenges of public health leadership?

How does each of the leadership theories presented help you to develop your own understanding of public health leadership?

Comment

You may have identified the need to develop a clear vision or provide a focus for health improvement as the most important aspect of public health leadership, or you may have seen the ability to identify appropriate leadership styles as being key. Whatever your view, it is likely that you also identified that leadership is considerably more complex than the theories presented so far would suggest. Sometimes public health leadership is within an organisation, or involves enabling others to lead. At other times, public health leadership is across organisations and involves influencing others. Public health leadership is inevitably complex, with a focus on leading not only within but also across organisations. None of the perspectives on leadership discussed so far provide a clear sense of how leadership takes place when there are a number of leaders, or when leadership is across organisations and there is no formal relationship.

More recent approaches to leadership view it as a dynamic social process (Hosking, 1997; Wenger and Snyder, 2000) where different people take part and play different roles at different times. Some of these approaches, such as *transformational leadership,* retain the notion of a central leader with followers, while others share a view of leadership where different people take part and play different roles at different times. Often, the term *distributed leadership* is used interchangeably with others such as *shared leadership*, *dispersed leadership*, *team leadership* and *democratic leadership*, and offers an understanding of how leadership takes place when there are a number of leaders, or when leadership is across organisations and there is no formal relationship. These are discussed in Chapter 2, and the implications for public health and health improvement considered.

Chapter summary

In this chapter we began by considering the relationship between leadership and management. Initially, three different ways of viewing the relationship between leadership and management were explored:

1. the view that leadership and management are the same thing;

2. the view that management is a component of leadership; and

3. the view that leadership is a subset of management.

Two further perspectives were presented, one which views the two concepts as distinct from one another, and an alternative view that sees an overlap between leadership and management. It was concluded that contemporary ideas about leadership and management share a consensus that leading and managing are different, although there is less clarity about whether they are distinct.

A range of more traditional approaches to leadership (trait, style or behavioural, situational and contingency theories) was presented, and the idea of emotional intelligence as key differentiator between average and outstanding performance as a leader was introduced. The chapter concludes by arguing that leadership for public health is complex, and suggests that more recent ideas viewing leadership as a social process might offer a greater understanding of how leadership takes place when there are a number of leaders, or when leadership is across organisations and there is no formal relationship. Chapter 2 explores these in more detail.

GOING FURTHER

Grint, K (ed.) (1997) *Leadership: Classical, Contemporary and Critical Approaches.* Oxford: Oxford University Press.
This is a useful discussion of classical, traditional and more recent approaches to leadership.

Kouzes, JM and Posner, BZ (1995) *The Leadership Challenge.* San Francisco, CA: Jossey-Bass.

This updated edition offers a presentation of leadership based on a framework for leadership development.

Van Maurik, J (2001) *Writers on Leadership*. London: Penguin.
This book provides an overview of key writers on leadership in the twentieth century.

Sadler, P (1997) *Leadership*. London: Kogan Page.
This book provides an introduction to the topic of leadership for people with some background in management or the social sciences. Chapters look at the nature of leadership, leadership and management, leadership qualities, leader behaviour, styles of leadership, recruiting and selecting future leaders, the developing process, cultural differences and diversity, role models and the 'new leadership'.

chapter 2

Leadership as a Social Process

Vicki Taylor

Meeting the Public Health Competences

This chapter will help you to evidence the following competences for public health (Public Health Skills and Career Framework):

- Level 5(2) Lead on discrete areas of work;
- Level 5(d) Knowledge of various leadership styles;
- Level 5(e) Knowledge of the difference between management and leadership;
- Level 6(a) Knowledge of the models and principles of leadership and their application;
- Level 7(b) Understanding of the models and principles of leadership and their potential use in improving population health and wellbeing;
- Level 8(1) Lead on improving population health and wellbeing within and/or across organisations;
- Level 8(2) Engage and lead a group to influence positively the population's health and wellbeing;
- Level 8(a) Understanding of the models and principles of leadership and their potential use in improving and protecting health and wellbeing and in motivating colleagues and partners;
- Level 8(f) Understanding of basic management models and theories associated with motivation and leadership.

This chapter will also assist you in demonstrating the following National Occupational Standards for public health:

- Provide leadership for your team (M&L_B5);
- Provide leadership in your area of responsibility (M&L_B6);
- Lead others in improving health and wellbeing (PHP45);
- Develop and sustain cross-sectoral collaborative working for health and wellbeing (PHS09);
- Provide leadership for your organisation (M&L_B7).

In addition, this chapter will be useful in demonstrating Standard 11 of the Public Health Practitioner Standards:

Standard 11. Work collaboratively with people from teams and agencies other than one's own to improve health and wellbeing outcomes – demonstrating:

a. awareness of personal impact on others;

b. constructive relationships with a range of people who contribute to population health and wellbeing;
c. awareness of:

i. principles of effective partnership working;
ii. the ways in which organisations, teams and individuals work together to improve health and wellbeing outcomes;
iii. the different forms that teams might take.

Overview

In Chapter 1 it was suggested that more recent ideas that view leadership as a social process might offer a greater understanding of public health leadership. Public health professionals are regularly required to lead initiatives to improve health at a local level. As mentioned previously, often this leadership involves a number of leaders, or is across organisations and where there is no formal relationship. This chapter draws on approaches to leadership that view leadership as a social process, and explores the nature of public health leadership.

The activities in this chapter will focus on:

- exploring a range of models of leadership that view it as a dynamic social process;
- appreciating the strengths and weaknesses of different approaches to leadership and their potential use in improving population health and wellbeing;
- understanding that leadership can be vested in different people at different times;
- exploring what is meant by public health leadership and the nature of leadership across organisational boundaries and systems.

This chapter uses theory, tools and case studies to explore leadership as a dynamic social process. After reading this chapter you will be able to:

- identify a range of models and definitions of leadership as a social process;
- appreciate the strengths and weaknesses of different approaches to leadership;
- identify the key challenges for public health leadership, and develop an understanding of public health leadership and what it entails.

Introduction

Leadership to improve public health is a complex process requiring leadership across organisations and an ability to engage with a wide range of people and organisations. Recent approaches to leadership that view it as a dynamic social process (Hosking, 1997; Wenger and Snyder, 2000), where different people take part and play different roles at different times, are particularly useful in understanding how public health leadership takes place when there are a number of leaders, or when leadership is across organisations and there is no formal hierarchy. Some of these approaches, such as *transformational leadership*, retain the notion of a central leader with followers, while others share a more elastic view of leadership where different people take part, playing different roles at different times. The latter is often referred to as *distributed*, *shared* or *dispersed leadership*, and is often used interchangeably with one another (Turnbull James, 2011).

Transformational leadership

In the last decade, transformational leadership has gained a degree of momentum across the public sector in the UK. Leadership frameworks developed for the police, National Health Service (NHS), schools and local government are based on this concept (see for example, the NHS Leadership Qualities Framework, the Police Integrated Competency Framework and the School Leadership Model).

Burns (1978), who was one of the first to put forward the concept of transformational leadership, argued that it was possible to distinguish between transactional and transforming leaders. The former is based on legitimate authority between leaders and followers, and the relationship is based on mutual dependence and an exchange process (Northouse, 1997). The latter is based on the leader engaging with their followers. This occurs when leaders

> *broaden and elevate the interests of their employees, when they generate awareness and acceptance of the purposes and mission of the group, and when they stir their employees to look beyond their own self-interest for the good of the group.*
>
> (Bass, 1990, p21)

Gandhi is often cited as an example of a transformational leader who, through his example and thinking, became an inspiration for others. Transformational leaders such as Gandhi seek to appeal to their followers' *better nature and move them toward higher and more universal needs and purposes* (Bolman and Deal, 1997, p314). Such leadership involves a focus on change and the importance of developing a clear direction or vision (Fulop *et al.*, 2004). Transformational leaders literally transform the way that people see themselves and their organisation. Followers are emotionally engaged and do more than is expected. Plsek and Greenhalgh (2001) have commented on the relevance of such an approach for complex environments where change is the norm. Leading for health improvement seems to fit this well, given the complexity of the environment.

What's the evidence?

Alimo-Metcalfe and Alban-Metcalfe (2000) have been key players in the development of transformational leadership. In their study of leadership, they conducted a survey of managers in the NHS and local government, and comment on the 'staggering complexity' of the role of leadership in the NHS. They found that staff in the NHS said that the most important prerequisite for the leader in terms of role is what they can do for their staff. Other reported findings were that leadership is about engaging others as partners, developing and achieving a shared vision and enabling others to lead. Being sensitive to the needs of a range of stakeholders (both internal and external to the organisation) and the ability to create *connectedness – joined-up thinking, even* (Alimo-Metcalfe and Alban-Metcalfe, 2000, pp27–9). They identify the following key factors of successful leaders:

- concern for others;
- approachability;
- encouraging questioning and promoting change;
- integrity;
- charisma;
- intellectual ability;
- the ability to communicate, set direction, unify and manage change.

Bass and Avolio (1994) suggest that transformational leaders display behaviours associated with five styles:

1. idealised behaviours – living one's ideals;

2. inspirational motivation – inspiring others;

3. intellectual stimulation – stimulating others;

4. individualised consideration – support, coaching and development;

5. idealised attributes – respect, trust and faith.

The behaviours associated with each of these five styles is set out below in more detail.

Behaviours associated with transformational styles

Idealised behaviours involve:

- Talking about their most important values and beliefs.
- Specifying the importance of having a strong sense of purpose.
- Considering the moral and ethical consequences of decisions.
- Championing exciting new possibilities.
- Talking about the importance of trusting each other.

Inspirational motivation involves:

- Talking optimistically about the future.
- Talking enthusiastically about what needs to be achieved.
- Articulating a compelling vision of the future.
- Expressing confidence that goals will be achieved.
- Taking a stand on controversial issues.

Intellectual stimulation involves:

- Appraising critical assumptions.
- Seeking different perspectives when solving problems.
- Suggesting new ways of looking at how to undertake tasks.
- Getting others to contribute to problem-solving from different angles.
- Encouraging non-traditional ways of thinking.
- Encouraging challenging thinking.

Individual consideration requires:

- Spending time teaching and coaching.
- Treating others as individuals.
- Considering others as having different needs, abilities and aspirations.
- Listening attentively to others.
- Promoting self-development.

Idealised attributes involve:

- Instilling pride in others for being associated with them.
- Going beyond self-interest for the good of the group.
- Acting in ways that build others' respect.
- Displaying a sense of power and competence.
- Making personal sacrifices for the benefit of others.
- Reassuring others that obstacles will be overcome.

Source: Bass and Avolio (1994)

Another useful way of thinking about transformational leadership is to consider it as leading for change, which is at the heart of leading for health improvement. The first step is in developing or creating a vision and demonstrating commitment to that vision. The second step is concerned with communicating the vision and engaging others in this process. The third step is implementing the vision, reorganising and building new ways of working. Tichy and Ulrich refer to this as *creation of a vision*, *mobilisation of commitment* and *institutionalisation of change* (1984, pp63–4) technically, culturally and politically. Ensuring that this takes place requires a consideration of what is happening at an emotional level and an understanding of what individuals are experiencing. The key skills of transformational leaders are in steering the vision and making things happen at all levels. This has some similarity with the eight-step approach to change proposed by Kotter (1995, 1996), which is discussed in Chapter 9.

ACTIVITY 2.1

Look back at the behaviours (identified by Bass and Avolio) and the key factors (identified by Alimo-Metcalfe and Alban-Metcalfe) as being important for transformational leadership.

How might these provide a framework for public health leadership?

What might be the relative strengths and weaknesses of a transformational leadership approach?

Comment

Developing a vision on how to improve health and inspiring others is central to public health leadership, and congruent with the enabling aims of much public health work. Working in partnership with others, within and across organisations and providing strategic direction, is at the core of the vision of public health leadership set out in the White Paper, *Healthy Lives, Healthy People: Our Strategy for Public Health in England* (Department of Health, 2010b, p51). The role of the director of public health is viewed as transforming the agenda to focus attention on protecting and improving the health of the local population.

One important criticism of transformational leadership is a perceived over-reliance on the leader and an apparent return to an almost 'heroic' view of leadership, with a focus on the leader at the expense of followers. The potential to develop dependency on the leader has led to a shift in focus on alternative models of leadership as a social process, where different people take part and play different roles at different times.

Leadership as a social process

Martin *et al.* (2010, p43) note the interdependence between leaders and followers and draw attention to the active participation of both parties. Leaders cannot exist without followers, and for any leader to be effective there needs to be a collective and shared view of the direction of change, as well as willingness to engage in the process. In considering leadership as a social process, attention becomes focused on different roles at different times and the notion of leadership as interaction. From this perspective there can be more than one leader and any member of a group can make leadership contributions.

Credited with advancing the idea of leadership as a social process, Kouzes and Posner (1987, 2007) identified a series of practices used by effective leaders at all levels. They were interested in how leaders led when they were at their best. From their research, involving more than 10,000 leaders, five practices of successful leaders who could be found at all levels of the organisation were identified:

Five practices identified by Kouzes and Posner

Challenging the process (status quo)

Leaders seek out opportunities to challenge the status quo, finding innovative ways of doing things, experimenting and taking risks. These leaders recognise that other people have good ideas, and encourage innovation and creativity from others. Importantly, they operate a no-blame culture in order to avoid stifling innovation. They encourage everyone to learn from experience and encourage people to try things out.

Inspiring a shared vision

Leaders have the ability to create a vision of the future and the confidence to make it happen. Importantly, such leaders are able to gain 'buy-in' from others and to develop a shared vision.

Enabling others to act

Leadership is a team effort, and support and assistance are required from everyone involved. Power is not kept, but given away. There is a belief in developing greater discretion, authority and information among others.

Leadership builds on trust and confidence and enables change. This in turn fosters collaboration and enables others.

Modelling the way

Leaders set an example through behaviour that gains respect. They are consistent and fair. Their style of planning and control is by continuous concentration on producing small wins that develop confidence. In this way, they show that even the biggest challenges can be met by hard work, perseverance and attention to detail. They create standards of excellence and set the example for others to follow. They are adept at unravelling bureaucracy and creating opportunities for success.

Encouraging the heart

Maintaining enthusiasm is a key task of the leader, because people can become tired, frustrated and disenchanted. Leaders harness and develop enthusiasm in others. As Kouzes and Posner put it, *Leaders encourage the hearts of their constituents to carry on* (1995, p14).

What is important about this approach is the recognition that leadership can be vested in anyone and at all levels. Power, responsibility and decision-making is not vested in one person but shared within a group, and leadership is constructed increasingly as a dynamic process (Martin *et al.*, 2010). Developing effective leadership processes within (and across) organisations becomes the key challenge.

ACTIVITY 2.2

Think about a public health initiative that you know well or in which you are involved.

Can you identify examples where the status quo was challenged?

How might you go about inspiring a shared vision? Can you think of examples where this was achieved?

What would be involved in enabling others to act? How might you encourage motivation and enthusiasm so that others want to keep going?

If you were asked to lead on an initiative to improve health and wellbeing, how might you use any of these practices? What would be involved?

How can you design processes to enhance effective leadership within this public health initiative?

Comment

You might have identified the need to find ways to develop the leadership skills of all those involved in health improvement and public health initiatives. This could include enabling others to lead on specific initiatives, creating a shared vision of the public health initiative using metaphors, or more simply by facilitating the process. Visualising success and getting others to see this vision is also a key challenge. Inspiring others to act and supporting ideas that others propose are central leadership activities.

Martin *et al.* suggest that leadership will be increasingly understood as *a dynamic process that includes and impacts upon people and progresses with a particular purpose* (2010, p44), where power, responsibility and decision-making are shared. This seems particularly applicable to public health leadership, where collaboration between and across organisations and the development of joint initiatives are critical to bringing about improvements in health. The King's Fund report, *The Future of Leadership and Management in the NHS: No More Heroes* (The King's Fund and Rowling, 2011), concluded that the *NHS needs to move beyond the outdated model of heroic leadership to recognise the value of leadership that is shared, distributed and adaptive* (2011, p22). One of the recommendations is that the NHS needs leadership across NHS boundaries into social care, local government, the voluntary sector and the wide variety of other agencies with which it interacts, and without whose co-operation it will not achieve its primary objectives. This is at the heart of public health and is increasingly important in achieving health improvement for all. A conceptualisation of leadership that is 'shared' and 'distributed', as identified in the King's Fund report (The King's Fund and Rowling, 2011, p22), is likely to become increasingly appealing. As organisational responsibility for public health in England moves from the NHS into local authorities, at the same time retaining responsibility for leading on health improvement across organisations and systems, the requirement for public health leadership to be an embedded quality of the system is becoming more critical.

Shared and distributed leadership

Turnbull James notes that the terms *dispersed, devolved, democratic, distributive, collaborative, collective, co-operative, concurrent, co-ordinated, relational and co-leadership* (2011, p6) have all been used to describe leadership in the twenty-first century. This type of leadership differs in that it recognises the involvement of *multiple actors* who take up leadership roles and, importantly, share leadership by working collaboratively (2011, p4). He also notes that the terms 'shared' and 'distributed' leadership are by far the most commonly used. While most writers seem to use these two terms interchangeably, Turnbull James makes a distinction between them. Drawing on the shared and distributed models of leadership that have been influential in the development of leadership in UK schools, he characterises shared leadership as involving *multiple entities* (2011, p6) and with it, collective influence. Writing on community leadership, Doyle and Smith (2009) refer to shared leadership, where leadership is vested in different people at different times depending on the position and skills they have and the leadership requirements (see Chapter 6 for a more detailed discussion).

'Distributed' leadership involves practices within and across the organisation (and presumably across organisations) and an associated capacity for collective action (Turnbull James, 2011, p7). Unlike shared leadership, this focuses attention on practices in and across organisations rather than on the leader. Elsewhere, distributed leadership has been described as the idea of *thinking about leadership as a quality of the whole organization, network or system* (Hartley *et al.*, 2008, p12). In direct contrast to those models, which advocate leadership from the top, distributed leadership places it at all levels of an organisation. From this perspective, each person is considered a leader. The ability to influence others and to carry them with them is central, as is a leader's relationship with others. Leadership becomes a collective enterprise, based on a premise of interactions between many leaders rather than the actions of an individual leader. A leader may not have formal power, and groups may have more than one leader. What is important about this approach is the recognition that leadership can be vested in anyone and at all levels. Power, responsibility and decision-making is not vested in one person, but shared within a group, and leadership is increasingly constructed as a dynamic process (Martin *et al.*, 2010). Developing effective leadership processes within (and across) organisations becomes *the* central challenge. Table 2.1 compares the features of shared and distributed (and adaptive) leadership.

Table 2.1 Features of shared and distributed leadership

Shared leadership	*Distributed and adaptive leadership*
Identified by the quality of people's interactions rather than on their position	Identified by the quality of leadership practices
Leadership is evaluated by how people are working together	Leadership is evaluated by considering the quality of practices across the system, network and organisation
Leadership comprises multiple entities, and with it, collective influence	Leadership consists of practices within and across the organisation(s) and an associated capacity for collective action
People are interdependent – all are active participants in the process of leadership	Practices are interdependent – the focus is on practices for leadership Individuals interact, creating a reciprocal interdependency between their actions
Communication is crucial, with a stress on conversation	Leadership practice is viewed as a product of interactions The interactions between people and their situation are critical in understanding leadership practice
Shared leadership values democratic processes, honesty and shared ethics – it seeks a common good	Distributed leadership is first and foremost about leadership practice rather than leaders or their roles, functions, routines and structures

Source: Adapted from Doyle and Smith (2009), Spillane (2005) and Turnbull James (2011)

ACTIVITY 2.3

What do you understand by the phrase 'public health leadership'?

What do you see as the most important aspects of public health leadership?

How does each of the leadership theories presented in this chapter help you to develop your understanding of public health leadership?

Comment

You may have identified that public health leadership is complex and involves leadership across and within organisations. Public health leaders are seen as having a central role in developing a vision for improving health and influencing others to achieve this vision. This might suggest a transformational leadership approach.

Strategic leadership that seeks to join up the public health agenda, across and within organisations, is central to the development of any public health vision to improve health and wellbeing. Public health leaders also need to balance many and sometimes conflicting factors and influences, and to work to develop a common agenda across organisations. This requires an ability to engage effectively with a wide range of people and organisations and manage a range of diverse perspectives. Leadership without authority is increasingly common as multi-agency programmes and initiatives are announced, set up and driven through. Shared leadership has a number of attributes that may be applicable to leadership for health improvement, as does distributed leadership. There is general agreement that leadership is a key element of public health work; however, the nature of leadership and what constitutes public health leadership remain open to wider debate.

Leading to improve health: public health leadership

Writing about leadership development in 1997, Catford notes that *there is an absolute paucity of research on what makes good public health leaders and how leadership can be strengthened* (Catford, 1997, p2). He raises questions about the transferability of much of leadership theory (which is based primarily on private corporate organisations) to the public sector and, in particular, to health promotion; also, about the nature of leadership to improve health. He suggests three different roles for public health leaders: as *creators of vision and strategy*, *managers of perception and meaning* and *facilitators of organisational effectiveness* (Catford, 1997, p4), and asks whether a theory of public health leadership can be created. Since then, others have commented on the need to develop a greater understanding of public health leadership. Carr *et al.* (2009, p206) note the limited literature on public health leadership and leadership development. While there seems to be agreement that it involves multiple professional groups, and that shared leadership is the current dominant discourse, there remains a lack of agreement on leadership for health improvement.

The development of a national strategy for public health leadership in the UK demonstrates recognition of the importance of leadership skills in achieving public health outcomes. This strategy (for public health leadership) was based on the development of a *network of individuals across the NHS and partner organisations, skilled in the areas of health improvement* (Rao, 2006). Transformation leadership was central to this strategy, although it is evident that ideas on shared leadership also have been influential. In England, two distinctly different approaches to leadership development were supported: the first aimed to develop individuals' capabilities as leaders (National Public Health Leadership Programme); and the second had a focus on individual leaders and a more collaborative whole system approach (Leadership for Health Improvement Programme). In 2002, the Institute for Public Health in Ireland launched an all-Ireland public health leadership programme (Leadership for Building a Healthy Society). The vision was to develop a network of leaders working collaboratively and creatively to build a healthy society and tackle health inequalities. The Scottish public health leadership programme, based on the Leadership for Health Improvement Programme, considers approaches across networks and systems using a model of distributed leadership (Carr *et al.*, 2009, p213).

Case study: Public Health Leadership Programme in the UK

The National Public Health Leadership Programme

This was developed in recognition of the importance of leadership skills in achieving public health.

The programme objectives were to:

- *Ensure that public health considerations are included in decisions concerning health and social policy at all levels within the NHS and other relevant organisations*
- *Foster better understanding of how leadership skills in people and organisations can improve health*
- *Identify and support the development of self-awareness and personal leadership styles and offer additional skills*
- *Promote strong multi-disciplinary and cross-sectoral working for health*
- *Develop a network of peers committed to shared learning and improving population health.*

(Leading for Health, National Public Health Leadership Programme 2008 invitation letter)

Leadership for Health Improvement Programme

The programme focused on the interlocking spheres of public health delivery systems, public health leadership and leadership for health improvement, underpinned by principles of building whole system relationships and understanding and using improvement methods (Figure 2.1).

Leadership for Health Improvement Programme in Scotland

In Scotland the Leadership for Health Improvement Programme, based on the Leadership for Health Improvement Programme in England, focuses on the development of those involved in health improvement. It is firmly based on a model of distributed leadership and linked to the Scotland Leadership Development Framework 'Delivery Through Leadership'.

Leadership for Building a Healthy Society

The strategy of the Institute of Public Health in Ireland is to strengthen leadership for public health and to help develop leadership capability among people who are working to build a healthy society on the island of Ireland.

In 2002, the Institute launched the leadership programme, Leadership for Building a Healthy Society. The vision for the programme was to develop a network of leaders who work collaboratively and creatively to build a healthy society and tackle health inequalities.

(*Source*: **www.inispho.org.uk/iphwork/buildingpublichealthcapacity/ leadership**; last accessed September 2011)

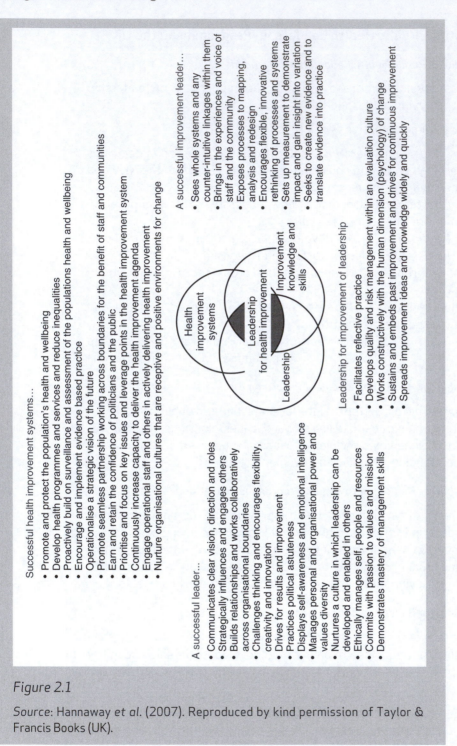

Successful health improvement systems...

- Promote and protect the population's health and wellbeing
- Develop health programmes and services and reduce inequalities
- Proactively build on surveillance and assessment of the populations health and wellbeing
- Encourage and implement evidence based practice
- Operationalise a strategic vision of the future
- Promote seamless partnership working across boundaries for the benefit of staff and communities
- Earn and retain the confidence of politicians and the public
- Prioritise and focus on key issues and leverage points in the health improvement system
- Continuously increase capacity to deliver the health improvement agenda
- Engage operational staff and others in actively delivering health improvement
- Nurture organisational cultures that are receptive and positive environments for change

A successful leader...

- Communicates clear vision, direction and roles
- Strategically influences and engages others
- Builds relationships and works collaboratively across organisational boundaries
- Challenges thinking and encourages flexibility, creativity and innovation
- Drives for results and improvement
- Practices political astuteness
- Displays self-awareness and emotional intelligence
- Manages personal and organisational power and values diversity
- Nurtures a culture in which leadership can be developed and enabled in others
- Ethically manages self, people and resources
- Commits with passion to values and mission
- Demonstrates mastery of management skills

A successful improvement leader...

- Sees whole systems and any counter-intuitive linkages within them
- Brings in the experiences and voice of staff and the community
- Exposes processes to mapping, analysis and redesign
- Encourages flexible, innovative rethinking of processes and systems
- Sets up measurement to demonstrate impact and gain insight into variation
- Seeks to create new evidence and to translate evidence into practice

Leadership for improvement of leadership

- Facilitates reflective practice
- Develops quality and risk management within an evaluation culture
- Works constructively with the human dimension (psychology) of change
- Sustains and embeds past improvement and drives for continuous improvement
- Spreads improvement ideas and knowledge widely and quickly

Figure 2.1

Source: Hannaway *et al.* (2007). Reproduced by kind permission of Taylor & Francis Books (UK).

One of the common features across all of these public health leadership development programmes is a focus on the development of leadership across networks and partnerships. Exercising external influence through partnerships and networks is important for public health and central to leadership for health improvement. Despite this, the idea of leadership across networks of organisations is one that has received little attention in the leadership literature until recently.

Looking at leadership in multi-sectoral organisations, Armistead *et al.* (2007, p221) found no obvious consensus on the essential nature of leadership in partnership. They comment on the challenges to leadership, noting that these are *compounded by the well-documented complexities of partnership working where there is a premium on the ability to influence and lead across a number of different organizations and organizational cultures* (2007, p216). Hartley *et al.* (2008) comment on the leadership challenges of working in networks and partnerships, because *leadership is generally fragile in conditions of diffuse power* (2008, p18). Denis *et al.* (2001) explore the strategic challenge for leaders in contexts where there are diverse interests and priorities within and between partners, and where leadership roles are shared, objectives are divergent and power is diffuse. They draw attention to four key characteristics of leadership in networks and partnerships, that it is collective, action-oriented, dynamic and supra-organisational (Denis *et al.*, 2001, p828; Hartley *et al.*, 2008, pp104–5).

Summary of key characteristics of leadership in networks and partnerships

Collective – many leadership contributions and different types of contributions;

Action/process-oriented – focusing on actions such as mobilising others and influencing;

Dynamic – leadership roles evolve continuously, with different power relationships at different times;

Supra-organisational – leadership roles and influences are beyond organisational boundaries and are complex.

Source: Adapted from Denis *et al.* (2001) and Hartley *et al.* (2008)

ACTIVITY 2.4

Think about a health improvement partnership that you know well, or in which you have been involved.

Who led this partnership?

Can you identify more than one leader in the partnership?

Do any of the key characteristics of leadership in networks and partnerships identified above apply to your experience?

Comment

There is increasing recognition of the challenge of leading partnerships and net-works. Much public health and health improvement is complex and requires leader-ship across and within organisations and at many levels. Recent work undertaken to identify how leadership happens in such contexts will provide a greater under-standing of the leadership challenges involved.

In this chapter a number of approaches to leadership have been discussed, however, it is inevitable that many have been omitted. There are many other ideas about leadership: for example, community leadership (see Chapter 6) and the theory of adaptive change and leadership (Heifetz, 1994; Heifetz and Laurie, 1997). More recently, the development of complexity leadership theory, based on complex sys-tems thinking and emphasising the dynamics of social networks, may have much to offer in developing a greater understanding of the particular aspects of leadership in the context of partnerships, together with further research on leadership in networks and partnerships.

Chapter summary

In this chapter we began by considering the complexity of leadership to improve health, and drew on approaches to leadership that view leadership as a social proc-ess. Common to these approaches is the recognition that leadership is a dynamic process where different people take part and play different roles at different times. Transformational leadership and the nature of public health leadership were explored. The interdependence between leaders and followers, and the notion of leadership as interaction, led to a discussion of shared and distributed leadership, before returning to consider public health leadership in more detail.

The development of a national strategy for public health leadership in the UK was seen as demonstrating recognition of the importance of leadership skills in achiev-ing public health outcomes. Transformational leadership is central to this strategy, although it is evident that ideas on shared leadership also have been influential.

Moving on to consider the public health leadership development programmes that have been established in the UK, it became apparent that a focus on the develop-ment of leadership across networks and partnerships was a common theme. This idea of leadership across networks of organisations is one which has received more attention recently, and it is suggested that the development of complex-ity leadership theory, emphasising the dynamics of social networks, may offer a greater understanding in the future of public health leadership across and within partnerships.

GOING FURTHER

Pearce, C and Conger, JA (2003) *Shared Leadership: Reframing the Hows and Whys of Leadership.* London: Sage.
This book provides a clear and informed review of the development of shared leadership as a paradigm. It addresses conceptual, methodological and practical issues for shared leadership in its endeavour to advance greater understanding of shared leadership, practice implications and shape directions for the future.

Hunter, D (ed.) (2007) *Managing for Health.* London: Routledge.
This book provides a clear exploration of the challenges for public health and health improvement, and explores the management challenge in public health. The key issues addressed by this book include the concept of managing for health or public health management, the importance of public health management, the skills and frameworks required of managers and practitioners working in health systems, and implications for training and development.

Armistead, C, Pettigrew, P and Aves, S (2007) Exploring leadership in multi-sectoral partnerships. *Leadership,* 3: 211–30.
This article explores key aspects of leadership in the context of multi-sectoral partnerships. In asking the question: 'How do managers experience and perceive leadership in such partnerships?', the study contributes to the debate on whether leadership in a multi-sectoral partnership context differs from that within a single organisation. It concludes that practising managers working in complex partnerships perceive leadership in partnerships to be more complex than in single organisations, but notes that there is no consensus on the nature of leadership.

Hazy, JK, Goldstein, JA and Lichtenstein, BB (2007) *Complex Systems Leadership: New Perspectives from Complexity Science on Social and Organisational Effectiveness.* Mansfield, MA: ISCE Publishing.
This volume brings together ideas on leadership and complexity, putting forward the argument that leadership can be enacted through any interaction in an organisation. Leadership is viewed as an emergent phenomenon within complex systems. The chapters in the volume are based on an understanding of the science underlying complexity and complex adaptive systems, offering new insights about leadership.

chapter 3

Working In and With Organisations
Vicki Taylor

Meeting the Public Health Competences

This chapter will help you to evidence the following competences for public health (Public Health Skills and Career Framework):

- Level 5(1) Collaborate with others effectively to improve population health and wellbeing;
- Level 5(3) Identify and influence other people and agencies in own area of work to improve population health and wellbeing;
- Level 5(5) Promote the value of population health and wellbeing and the reduction of inequalities in various teams or agencies *[an understanding of organisations is central to this competence]*;
- Level 5(j) Awareness of how people can help to build capacity and capability in the system overall *[an understanding of organisations is central to this competence]*;
- Level 6(5) Promote the value of health and wellbeing and the reduction of inequalities across settings and agencies *[an understanding of organisations is central to this competence]*;
- Level 7(2) Engage and influence others in and beyond own organisation to improve population health and wellbeing *[an understanding of organisations is central to this competence]*;
- Level 8(1) Lead on improving population health and wellbeing within and/or across organisations *[an understanding of organisations is central to this competence]*;
- Level 8(2) Engage and lead a group to influence positively the population's health and wellbeing *[an understanding of organisations is central to this competence]*;
- Level 8(b) Understanding of how various organisational cultures can influence the outcomes of collaborative work;
- Level 8(c) Understanding of the roles that various organisations, agencies, individuals and professionals play and the influence they may have on health and health inequalities.

This chapter will also assist you in demonstrating the following National Occupational Standards for public health:

- Map the environment in which your organisation operates (M&L_B2);
- Develop productive working relationships with colleagues and stakeholders (M&L_D2);

- Develop and sustain cross-sectoral collaborative working for health and wellbeing (PHS10);
- Develop the culture of your organisation (M&L_B9).

In addition, this chapter will be useful in demonstrating Standard 11 of the Public Health Practitioner Standards:

Standard 11. Work collaboratively with people from teams and agencies other than one's own to improve health and wellbeing outcomes – demonstrating:

b. constructive relationships with a range of people who contribute to population health and wellbeing;
c. awareness of:

    i. principles of effective partnership working;
    ii. the ways in which organisations, teams and individuals work together to improve health and wellbeing outcomes;
    iii. the different forms that teams might take.

Overview

This chapter will help you to consider what organisations are, why they exist and how they work, and to consider the implications for public health and health improvement. In this chapter we will consider the relationship between an organisation and its external environment before focusing on internal organisational structure and culture. We will review some classical ideas about organisations, and consider more recent emerging organisational forms and the implications for public health. In addition, organisational mission and purpose and how this is articulated will be explored. Finally, we will consider some key challenges for public health related to working in and with organisations, and look at the implications for public health and health improvement initiatives.

The activities in this chapter will focus on:

- exploring your own values and the values of your organisation;
- understanding organisational and personal objectives and the purpose of your organisation;
- appreciating the external environment and external influences on your organisation;
- completing a systems map of your organisation, showing where the boundaries lie and considering implications for your public health and health improvement work;
- understanding the organisational structure of your own and other organisations that you work with;
- clarifying the organisational culture in which you operate.

This chapter uses theory, tools and case studies to explore the nature of organisations.

After reading this chapter you will be able to:

- explain the purpose of organisations;
- be able to map the environment in which your organisation operates;
- identify a range of models and definitions of organisation, structure and culture;
- appreciate the strengths and weaknesses of different approaches to organisational structure and culture.

Key features of organisations

What is a public health organisation? On the surface this seems to be a straightforward question, but the term 'organisation' often means different things to different people. If you were to consider your organisation from the perspective of different members of staff – for example, a public health practitioner, director of finance, director of public health or chief executive – it is likely that each will have a different perception and definition of it. However, there are some key features that are common to all organisations.

- Organisations consist of people – these people often have some shared values and views about the purpose of the organisation.

- Organisations exist for a purpose – often, this is expressed as a hierarchy of purposes with a set of organisational goals and specific objectives.

- Organisations are affected and shaped by factors in the wider environment – such as changes in the economy, social trends and the political climate.

- Organisations exist in relationship with others – they may be large and complex or small and simple, the organisational boundaries clear or blurred.

- Organisations do not just happen, they are designed – organisations have some control over how they organise themselves to achieve their objectives.

- Organisations have distinct cultures.

Organisations consist of people

Think of the organisations that you know or those you have worked in: one thing they all have in common is that they consist of people who have some shared values and views about the purpose of the organisation. In turn, the organisational values are shaped by those people who make up the organisation and influenced by the wider world in which it functions. Martin *et al.* (2010) refer to societal, organisational, group and individual values in an attempt to consider the complex nature of, and potentially conflicting, values that are involved in working in health and social care. Societal values are those values that are shared at a societal level: for example, current government public health policy in England is based on working in partnership to promote responsibility for healthy lifestyle behaviours. This has as an underlying value of individual freedom, fairness and individual responsibility (Department of Health, 2010b). Nationally the NHS values of respect and dignity, commitment to quality of care, compassion, improving lives, purpose, working together and inclusion are expressed (Department of Health, 2010c).

At an organisational level, the organisation's values and beliefs might be expressed as *reducing inequalities and social exclusion, securing fair, fast access to a comprehensive range of services* and *increasing choice*. The values behind these include equity, fairness and choice. Within an organisation it is likely that there will be group or team values. Martin *et al.* (2010, p80) note that people from other organisations are being increasingly brought into an integrated service, and this may result in competing or conflicting sets of values. Differing sets of values also may exist within organisations, reflecting distinct professional backgrounds. For example, in a public health team the most important value might be that of equity, while a commissioning team within the same organisation might have choice as the most important value. These two values could be in conflict with one another.

At an individual level our values are based on our social background, upbringing, education, religious background and life experience, among others. Typically, these values will influence and be influenced by those of the group, organisation and society. One of the challenges is to understand the interplay between these different and potentially competing levels of values.

ACTIVITY 3.1

Think about those values that are important to you.

What is your most important value or belief?

What are the values held by your organisation?

Can you think of examples at work where your values have been incompatible with those of other individuals, groups or your organisation?

Comment

You may have found it difficult to identify your values, and where you were able to identify them, it is likely that not all will be consistent with one another. This is not that surprising and it is not necessarily a problem, as we can usually manage some degree of tension. Magnifying this to consider values at the group, organisational and societal levels highlights some of the challenges posed for public health and health improvement work.

Organisations exist for a purpose

All organisations need to have a clear sense of direction, ideally one that flows throughout the organisation. Often this sense of direction is expressed as a hierarchy of purposes (also referred to as the 'pyramid of purpose', see Figure 3.1), which has clear links to the organisational aims or goals, and to specific objectives and targets. At the top of the hierarchy is a description of why the organisation exists, then some broad statements about what the organisation is trying to do, and then, at a lower level in the hierarchy, more specific objectives and targets are stated, which set out how these activities are going to be done.

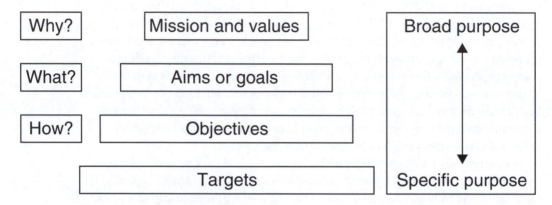

Figure 3.1 Hierarchy of purpose ('pyramid of purpose')

ACTIVITY 3.2

Think about the organisation in which you currently work.

Does it have a statement about the organisational purpose(s) or a mission statement?

If so, how explicit and how widely understood and agreed is it?

How does this statement (or its absence) affect your public health and health improvement work?

Are there clear organisational aims or goals?

How do the organisational (departmental and individual) objectives relate to these organisational goals?

How do your individual objectives fit with the overall organisational goals?

Comment

You might have concluded that your organisation has a clear mission statement and that there is good agreement about what it is. You also may have noted that your individual objectives relate clearly to departmental objectives, and that these in turn fit clearly into the overall goals of the organisation. Depending on how large or small the organisation is, the people within the organisation will shape and influence its overall purpose through the values they bring. These values will have an important influence on the organisational goals and how things get done. Hudson argues that it is the process of working together to develop a mission statement that can be *a powerful lever for increasing the organisation's effectiveness* (1999, p95). You might like to consider the significance of this for your own work.

The following extracts are some examples of mission statements from organisations such as the World Health Organization (WHO), Faculty of Public Health, UK Public Health Register and Action on Smoking and Health (ASH).

Case study: Examples of organisational mission statements

WHO

WHO is the directing and coordinating authority for health within the United Nations system. It is responsible for providing leadership on global health matters, shaping the health research agenda, setting norms and standards, articulating evidence-based policy options, providing technical support to countries and monitoring and assessing health trends.

In the 21st century, health is a shared responsibility, involving equitable access to essential care and collective defence against transnational threats.

(*Source*: www.who.int/about/en/; accessed 29 July 2011)

Faculty of Public Health

Our overarching mission is to promote and protect the health and well-being of everyone in society by playing a leading role in assuring an effective public health workforce, promoting public health knowledge and advocating for the very best conditions for good health.

We are guided by our three main charitable objectives, which are to:

- promote for the public benefit the advancement of knowledge in the field of public health;
- develop public health with a view to maintaining the highest possible standards of professional competence and practice;
- act as an authoritative body for the purpose of consultation and advocacy in matters of educational or public interest concerning public health.

Our vision
The world's population achieves and maintains its fullest potential for health and wellbeing.

What we do
To fulfil our role in standard setting and supporting the public health profession the Faculty of Public Health works in three key areas:

Education and standards
Professional affairs
Advocacy and policy contribution.
(*Source*: **www.fph.org.uk/our_mission**; accessed 29 July 2011)

UK Public Health Register

The UK Public Health Register is an independent regulator for public health professionals in the UK.

Our purpose is to protect the public by regulating public health professionals.

We do this by:

- working with partners, setting and promoting standards for admission to the register and for remaining on the register;
- dealing with registered specialists who fail to meet the necessary standards;
- publishing a register of competent professionals.
(*Source*: **www.publichealthregister.org.uk**; accessed 10 October 2011)

Action on Smoking and Health (ASH)

ASH was established in 1971 by the Royal College of Physicians. It is a campaigning public health charity that works to eliminate the harm caused by tobacco. We do not attack smokers or condemn smoking. The organisation is headed by the Chief Executive, Deborah Arnott, and governed by a Board of Trustees. The Duke of Gloucester is our patron.

While we aim to be innovative and agenda setting in our work, our policies are always evidence based and follow a dual approach:

Information and networking: To develop opinion and awareness about the 'tobacco epidemic'
Advocacy and campaigning: To press for policy measures that will reduce the burden of addiction, disease and premature death attributable to tobacco.

ASH works towards achieving four strategic priorities as outlined in our *Strategic Plan 2008–11*. They cover all areas of ASH's work, both in terms of current activities and future directions.
(*Source*: **www.ash.org.uk/about-ash**; accessed 29 July 2011)

The mission statement sets out why the organisation exists, what its aims are, who it is for and where it operates (i.e. locally, nationally, internationally). It enshrines the organisation's purpose and values. In some of the examples, values are stated explicitly and, in many cases, information on how the organisation works is provided.

ACTIVITY 3.3

Look at the mission statements of the key organisations that you work with in delivering health improvement.

In each case, can you identify why the organisation exists?

To what extent does the mission statement reflect a commitment to improving health?

What are the underlying values or principles?

What are the implications for your personal and organisational objectives?

What are the implications for your public health and health improvement work?

Comment

Public health professionals work in many different types of organisations, and often are required to deliver and develop initiatives that have an impact across more than one organisation. Given that much public health and health improvement takes place across organisations and within partnerships, you might like to consider how the mission statements of all those organisations who need to work together to improve health demonstrate a commitment to this objective.

Organisations are affected and shaped by factors in the wider environment

Public sector organisations, and public health organisations in particular, seem to have gone through endless change in the past decade. In fact, organisational change seems to be continuous, but what causes these changes? Organisations do not operate in a vacuum (Mullins, 2002; Buchanan and Huczynski, 2004) but continually interact with the external environment. An understanding of the external environment is particularly critical for public health managers because it provides a source of many threats and new opportunities as well as drivers for change. For example, the publication of *Healthy Lives, Healthy People* (Department of Health, 2010b) has had an enormous impact on the way in which public health is organised, with public health shifting from the NHS to local government.

Organisational effectiveness is dependent on successful management of the opportunities and threats presented by these external influences for change, together with the internal response to these challenges. This complex network can be represented by the following, commonly referred to as the 'three environments' model (Figure 3.2).

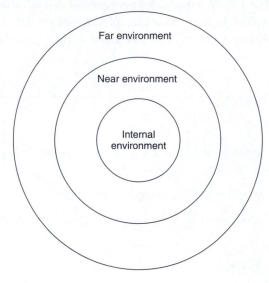

Figure 3.2 The three environments

The *far* external environment refers to factors that cannot be easily controlled or influenced directly from within the organisation. They include a wide range of political, environmental, social, technological, legal and economic factors. All organisations need to be aware of these external factors and respond to their impact.

The *near* external environment includes all those groups and organisations with whom the organisation interacts. These include local politicians, suppliers, organisations that are in partnership with the organisation and local interest groups. They cannot be controlled by the organisation, but they can be influenced.

The *internal* environment represents the organisation, its employees and resources. It is argued that the internal environment is one in which managers can exert control; however, the internal environment is also shaped and influenced by the near and far (external) environments (this will be discussed later in this chapter).

ACTIVITY 3.4

Using Table 3.1, identify the external factors which currently have an impact on or are influencing your organisation.

Table 3.1 PESTLE factors

PESTLE factor	Key features	Organisational impact
Political	Political direction, policies, ideology	
Economic	General state of the economy, salaries, disposable income, interest rates, taxation	
Social	Population demographics, public preferences, attitudes and behaviours, population profile	
Technological	Available technology, uses of technology (smartphones, text messaging, social media)	
Legal	Legislation through Acts, Bills and Orders (Wales) such as the Children and Young Persons (Protection from Tobacco) Act 1991, Public Health (Control of Disease) Act 1984, Health and Social Care Bill 2011, The Public Health Wales National Health Service Trust (Originating Capital) (Wales) Order 2011, Public Health (Scotland) Act 2008	
Environmental	Current and future thinking on environmental issues	

Comment

If you are working in public health or working to improve health, it is likely that you will have identified changes in the political climate and the introduction of new governmental policy as key factors. The publication of *Healthy Lives, Healthy People* (Department of Health, 2010b) set out a strategy for public health in England which has far reaching implications. Changing social problems and population demographics, new patterns of funding and legislation also have a significant impact.

Organisations exist in relationship with others

How an organisation defines its external environment depends on where it defines its organisational boundary. Some organisations do most things in-house and have large core structures, whereas others outsource a lot of activities to other organisations in order to carry out core activities in the organisation. The case study below illustrates the different boundaries of two public health organisations.

Case study: Two public health organisations and their boundaries

Public Health Carden and Health Improvement Bellen are both public health organisations with similar levels of funding and similar aims: namely, to promote health and wellbeing, and to reduce inequalities in health status. Each organisation prioritises enabling community development as well as advocacy for health improvement, and is committed to developing capacity and capability at a local level.

Public Health Carden has a staff of around ten, but carries out most of its health-promoting activity via a contract with a small health promotion team in the local NHS trust, and commissions a team of health promotion staff in the local authority. Much of the other work is carried out through a range of partner organisations, funded through a mix of grants and contracts. These include the Healthy Carden Cities team located in the voluntary sector, Carden Mental Health collaborative and the Carden Women's Health Group.

Health Improvement Bellen is an integral part of the public health team within Claremont. All staff are employed by the organisation, and all activities are carried out by these staff, together with a small number of partnerships that have been developed specifically to improve health. The boundaries for each organisation can represented using a systems map, as in Figure 3.3.

These two diagrams illustrate how the choice of where to set organisational boundaries affect what is located within the organisation. Boundaries are not fixed and can change in response to external pressures (for example, political changes that require organisational change, such as aforementioned recent move of public health from the NHS to local government).

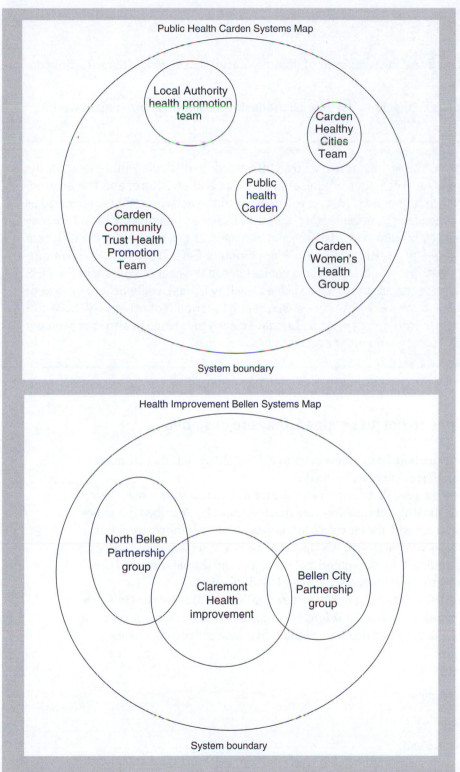

Figure 3.3 Systems maps of Public Health Carden and Health Improvement Bellen

ACTIVITY 3.5

Try to complete a systems map of your organisation, showing where the boundaries lie.

What are the implications for your public health and health improvement work?

Comment

Whether you found this activity straightforward or difficult will depend on the interactions between your organisation, its size and structure, and the environment in which it operates. Also, it will depend on the activities that are viewed as core activities for the organisation, and those seen as non-core. This in turn may be affected by factors in the external environment, as can be seen by the different configurations of health promotion. Many Primary Care Trusts (PCTs) have outsourced health promotion to other organisations in the near environment (i.e. NHS trusts, third-sector organisations such as Healthy Cities), while others have kept health promotion as a central core public health function. Yet others still have created social enterprise organisations, or have clearly identified health improvement units within local government organisations.

Organisations do not just happen, they are designed

In addition, organisational structure is determined by the decisions that are made about location, size, resources and so forth.

Weber (1947) argued that the most effective form of organisation is one where the roles and relationships of employees are clearly defined. He described this structure as a bureaucracy, with the idea of a *legal-rational authority* at the centre of this notion. This organisational structure is characterised by a belief that rules and legal order provide legitimacy for the authority of managers, and that it is designed like a machine in order to achieve organisational goals and objectives.

Mintzberg defined organisational structure (see Figure 3.4) as *the sum total of the ways in which it divides its labour into distinct tasks and then achieves coordination among them* (1979, p2). He proposed that all organisations consist of five components:

1   the strategic apex;

2   the operating core;

3   the middle line;

4   support staff and;

5   the technostructure (Mintzberg, 1983a).

Table 3.2 summarises the key features of each component.

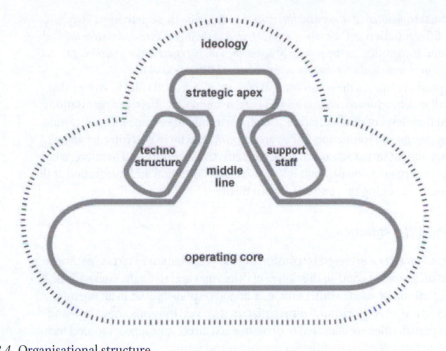

Figure 3.4 Organisational structure

Source: Mintzberg (1983a, p11)

Table 3.2 Five key components of an organisation

Strategic apex	Senior leadership – director of public health, chief executive and board members
Operating core	The people who do the fundamental work in the organisation
Middle line	The people who connect the strategic apex to the operating core – typically, departmental managers
Support staff	The people who directly support the work of those in the operating core
Technostructure	The technical staff whose work is required but not central to the operation of the organisation – an example might be public health information analysts

An organisational structure provides the framework to enable an organisation to divide and carry out the work of the organisation. The structure of an organisation underpins how it operates, and the 'rules' enable participation. Organisational structure provides a framework for allocating responsibilities and authority, and can be instrumental in establishing an organisation's identity. In an environment where there is increasing change and uncertainty, structure also can provide some sense of continuity.

The more complex an organisation, the more complex the processes for dividing up the work or tasks that need to be undertaken to achieve the organisational purpose, and for coordinating and integrating them. Lawrence and Lorsch (1967) coined the terms *differentiation* and *integration* to describe these activities. They defined differentiation as the *state of segmentation of the organisational system into sub-systems*, and integration as the *process of achieving unity of effort among various sub-systems in the accomplishment of the organisation's task* (1967, pp3–4).

Integration requires the co-ordination of people, tasks and roles to ensure that the overall task is achieved. Lawrence and Lorsch found that effective organisations increased their level of differentiation as their environment became more uncertain. However, greater differentiation brings greater scope for increased interdepartmental conflict and, in turn, increases the need for effective integration. Therefore, a key challenge for organisational design is to achieve differentiation and integration at the same time as managing the tension between them.

Achieving differentiation

Differentiation can be achieved by considering the organisation in terms of its tiers or hierarchies, span of control, the degree of delegation and so forth. These are all variables that can be used to differentiate tasks and responsibilities in an organisation at a vertical level. Horizontal differentiation involves decisions about how and where responsibilities are allocated to departments, directorates, geographical locations and so forth, leading to different organisational forms.

Vertical Differentiation

Span of control

This relates to the number of people reporting directly to a manager. Several factors will influence this, for example, the degree of interrelated work: where individuals are working on closely interrelated tasks, the job of co-ordination will be easier if they report to the same person.

Shape of hierarchy

A classic bureaucracy can be represented as a hierarchy with a number of layers of staff at different levels of seniority. Organisations with many levels are called 'tall', and those with few levels, 'flat'. Research by Pugh (1988) found that two-thirds of organisations had between five and eight levels of management.

Degree of centralisation

Centralised decision-making takes longer, as decisions have to be referred up the chain of command. Conversely, decisions are likely to be more consistent, with better control and clearer accountability. In addition to being quicker, decentralised decision-making provides more flexibility, is more responsive to local situations, and may sustain staff motivation, as they will feel greater ownership of their work.

Degree and type of specialisation

Jobs may be specialised because they require special knowledge, or because a complex task has been broken down into simpler elements.

Degree of job definition

In many organisations jobs are clearly and precisely defined, indicating exactly the postholder's responsibilities, authority and reporting line. This is central to the bureaucratic ideal, and has many advantages.

ACTIVITY 3.6

Look at your organisation and try to draw a chart to represent how the organisation is structured.

How many people report to each manager?

What is your span of control?

How many layers or levels of management are there?

Is your organisation tall or flat?

How much autonomy does each worker have?

Is authority centralised or decentralised?

Does your organisation employ functional experts for some tasks (for example, a finance department)?

How clear is the definition of jobs?

Do some of them overlap?

How many people do employees report to?

What are the implications of this?

Horizontal Differentiation

Functional structure

Differentiating on the basis of function is useful when people in functional departments need to communicate regularly with one another. For example, you may have a separate finance department or communications department. Although there is a need to communicate with all parts of the organisation, where the majority of the need is to communicate within a functional grouping, then the decision may be made to group people together. For example, all staff with a public health role may be grouped together as the public health directorate.

Product or service structure

People may be grouped on the basis of the product or service area. For example, staff within health and social care settings are often organised on the basis of the client group, older people's services, children and young people.

Geographic structure

Differentiating on the basis of geographical location is another way of dividing organisational tasks. For example, for a given public health team where the organisational structure is based on three distinct neighbourhoods, public health staff in location A would be based together with all other staff in the organisation who have a focus on location A. All staff whose work is based on location B would be grouped together, and so forth.

Project teams

These draw staff from across the organisation, often seconded on a full or part-time basis. A good example of this is where a specific team to reduce inequalities was set up in a unitary authority. Staff were drawn from across the unitary authority departments and seconded into the 'Inequalities' team.

Matrix structure

This represents a more permanent form of project structure, where people often have two reporting lines: one to the functional head, and one to the project head. Matrix structures can be difficult to manage, and having dual accountability can provide a challenge. Buchanan and Huczynski (2004) suggest that dual reporting can lead to ambiguity and conflict. Matrix structures can suffer from low responsiveness, slow decision-making and high levels of internal political conflict.

Networks

Increasingly, organisations need to look beyond their boundaries and many form networks or operate in partnerships with others. Some of these partnerships are informal, and others more formal with clear legislative frameworks. Whatever the arrangements, inter-organisational collaboration and partnership working introduce further complexity. (Chapter 4 looks at strategic partnerships and working across organisational boundaries in more detail, and highlights some of the potential benefits as well as costs of working in partnership.)

ACTIVITY 3.7

Looking back at Activity 3.5 and the organisational chart that you drew, together with the material on horizontal differentiation, which type of structure does your organisation have?

What are the pros and cons of this structure?

What changes would improve your organisation's structure?

Why do you think these changes are not implemented?

What organisational structure would be most effective for public health and health improvement work? Why?

What would need to happen to make this possible?

Comment

If your organisation is large then it is likely that you identified your organisation as having a functional structure. A smaller organisation is likely to require less differentiation and may not fit any of these organisational forms. Friedman (2011, drawing on Charnes and Smith Tewksbury, 1993) discusses five organisational designs for public health work: Functional, Divisional, Matrix, Parallel and Program, which are similar to the organisational forms discussed here. He concludes that organisational design is a dynamic process dependent on the vision of public health leaders who are aware of the environment in which they are operating, and that in public health settings the choice of organisational design is particularly important. However, he counsels against *falling into the trap of thinking there is no one best organization design* (2011, p31).

Achieving integration

Integrating all of the activities and tasks that have been differentiated across the organisation as a whole is a challenge, and so mechanisms need to be developed and put in place. Mullins (2002) identifies four mechanisms for achieving integration, which are summarised in Table 3.3.

Setting goals and targets for different groups and enabling them to take responsibility is another important way to achieve integration. In addition, building 'slack' into an organisation can enable greater co-ordination, as can creating self-contained tasks. Given the importance of ensuring that information reaches those who need it in a timely manner in order to inform decision-making and so on, developing a system to ensure clear communications channels is paramount. Central co-ordination and direction across a complex organisation requires access to full information and an adequate picture of what is happening. Finally, developing and fostering lateral relations, enabling decisions to be made, is also important in

Table 3.3 Mechanisms for achieving integration

Mechanism	Comment
Policies, rules and procedures	All organisations have procedures for dealing with routine activities
	Common in bureaucratic organisations
Teamwork and mutual cooperation	More commonly used in smaller, organic structures
Formal committees and project teams	As increased differentiation develops, more integration is required
	Can be managed through more 'formal' methods and processes
Assigned 'integrators'	Useful to minimise or to help resolve problems of co-ordination and work programming between different departments

Source: Adapted from Mullins (2002)

achieving integration – particularly in highly differentiated organisations where there is some sort of matrix structure. Examples of these relations could be between team leaders, establishing focused task groups, management team meetings and integrated departments.

ACTIVITY 3.8

Which, if any, of these approaches are used to co-ordinate activities in your organisation?

Which could be developed to improve the flow of information?

Which of these mechanisms are formal or informal?

Comment

You probably identified that a range of mechanisms are used. Often, public health is managed across a number of different organisations, or through networks. This adds greater complexity to the challenges of differentiation and integration.

Organisations have distinct cultures

The ways of working and getting things done in an organisation, and taken-for-granted everyday actions and beliefs, are often referred to as 'organisational culture'. Sometimes this is manifested in the practices undertaken and the ways in which people carry out the work. Trice and Beyer (1984) suggest that culture is manifested in and through the symbols of organisations. Some of these (which they refer to as *high-profile symbols*) such as logos, mission statements and annual reports are more obvious. Others (*low-profile symbols*) include practices, communications, physical attributes (such as the way that offices are organised) and common languages. Table 3.4 gives some examples of categories of low-profile symbols.

Table 3.4 Categories of low-profile symbols

Categories	Examples
Practices – defined as rites, rituals and ceremonies	Practices for making tea or coffee
	Work group outings for meals or drinks
	Annual office party
	Doctor's ward round in a hospital
	Award night for 'salesperson of the year'
	Director's visit to a regional office
	Long-service award ceremonies
Communications – stories, myths, symbols	Stories told repeatedly by members of the organisation, which influence behaviour
Physical forms – organisational forms such as office layout and dress code	How offices are arranged
	Posters or artworks
	Accepted dress code
	Furniture, etc.
Common languages	The jargon that is used by an organisation and provides some of its identity, affecting the way that people respond to their work

Source: Adapted from Trice and Beyer (1984)

Case study: Teenage pregnancy partnership for Area X

Background

The teenage pregnancy partnership has existed for nine years in Area X, jointly chaired by the council and the PCT. It has always involved a wide range of people from different levels within their organisations. It has focused on discussing multi-agency action plans to reduce teenage conceptions and improve support for teenage parents in the area. The teenage pregnancy rate in the area is high and has not reduced in line with the national fall in teenage conceptions.

Purpose:
• to oversee the implementation of the teenage pregnancy strategy in the area;
• to advise the council and the PCT on the effective deployment of resources.

Partners involved:

- local authority children's services staff (youth service, education, Early Years, Connexions);
- local authority housing services staff (occasional attendees);
- PCT public health, health promotion, family planning, health visiting and school nursing;
- voluntary sector providers of support and advice for young people;
- school-based health centre workers.

ACTIVITY 3.9

The teenage pregnancy partnership is an example of a partnership to improve health that can be found in most areas. Looking at the members of this partnership (or one that you are more familiar with), think about the following questions.

How might each of the members of the partnership talk about health?

Is there a common understanding?

What jargon might be used by each of the different members of the partnership?

How might practices differ?

Now think about the characteristics of the organisational culture in which you operate.

Are there any high- or low-profile symbols that seem to be different at the organisational or departmental level?

If so, what are they, and why might the differences exist?

Comment

Exploring ideas about culture can be complex when applied to public health work, where many organisations come together to improve the health and wellbeing of the local population. It is likely that there will be different understandings of health and wellbeing and different ways of communicating this. You may have considered the differences in how each of these partners might perceive health, teenagers and pregnancy, or even in how they speak about them. Each member of the partnership belongs to an organisation, and each organisation has its own practices and rituals, jargon, ways of communicating and doing things – its own organisational culture. In the same way, within organisations there may be different practices, rituals and so forth, often referred to as sub-cultures.

There have been numerous attempts to define culture. Deal and Kennedy provide a succinct and simple definition of culture, as *the way things get done around here* (1982, p4). Deal and Kennedy argue that the biggest influence on the culture of an organisation is the environment in which it operates. They proposed that two key dimensions, risk (low–high) and feedback (quick–slow), shape organisational culture. The interplay between these dimensions makes up their model of corporate culture. The four types of culture they proposed are as follows.

1 *Tough-guy, macho* – quick feedback within the organisation, high-risk activities and decisions feature.

2 *Work hard, play hard* – quick feedback within the organisation, low-risk activities and decisions feature.

3 *Bet your company* – slow feedback within the organisation, high-risk activities and decisions feature.

4 *Process culture* – slow feedback within the organisation, low-risk activities and decisions feature.

Handy (1988) proposed that culture is a product of the shared rules of behaviour in organisations, and identified four distinct types of culture: power (or club), task, person and role cultures.

Power culture

Handy depicts a power (or club) culture as a web, in recognition that the key to the whole organisation sits in the centre, connected to and pulling the strings of an ever-widening network of intimates and influence. The organisation is likened to a club, enabling the decisions of those at the centre to be undertaken. Communication is between individuals rather than more formal forms of communication. A charismatic figure characterises the culture and personality is important. The culture relies heavily on individual response and commitment, and person–organisation fit is key, with a family feel to the organisation.

Task culture

Handy likened a task culture to a net in which groups are put together and assembled in different ways, depending on what needs to be done. The intersection of the nets represents the place where power and influence lie. Competent people who enjoy new challenges and are stimulated by joining different teams for different purposes often prefer a task culture. Co-ordinators and team leaders, rather than managers, are central figures. Information technology (IT) companies are often cited as an example of this culture.

Person culture

A person culture puts individuals and their interests first, and sees the organisation as a means to an end. Handy represented the person culture as a constellation of loosely clustered stars. A consulting partnership (and many virtual organisations) is typical of this type of culture.

Role culture

In a role culture, people have clearly delegated authorities within a highly defined structure. A role culture is represented by Handy as a building supported by pillars and columns, representing specific roles in keeping the building up. Interrelated roles formalise communications and systems and procedures typify this type of culture. Certainty, stability and regulation are important organisational values. Figure 3.5 illustrates these four culture types.

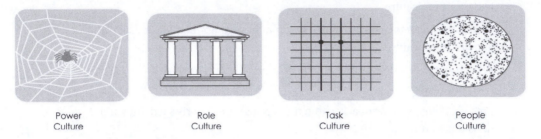

Power Culture   Role Culture   Task Culture   People Culture

Figure 3.5 Handy's four cultural types

Source: Handy (1993, pp183–90)

ACTIVITY 3.10

Using Deal and Kennedy's model of organisational culture, plot where you think the various sub-cultures sit within your organisation.

Think of a partnership you know well. Where would you place the culture of each of the organisations in the partnership on this model?

Now look at Handy's classification of culture. How would you describe the culture of your own organisation?

Comment

Often culture is seen as something that an organisation has. However, it is important to remember that culture is something that is created and shared by everyone within an organisation (or partnership), which develops and evolves over time.

Chapter summary

In this chapter we began by considering what a public health organisation is and introduced some key features common to all organisations. The people that make up organisations, and the values that they hold, were considered. The overall purpose of an organisation was explored and the mission statements of some key public health organisations presented. The impact of the external environments in which organisations operate, the influences of the internal environment and the relationship of the organisation with others led to a consideration of organisational boundaries, acknowledging that boundaries are not fixed and can change in response to external pressures.

Organisations do not just happen, they are designed; and organisational structure is determined by the decisions that are made about location, size, resources and so forth. A range of organisational structures were explored and it was noted that the more complex an organisation is, the more complex are its processes for dividing up the work or tasks that need to be undertaken to achieve the organisational purpose, and for coordinating and integrating these activities. Organisational ways of doing things, or culture, and the complexity of working together in partnerships where a number of organisational cultures collide, was seen as adding to the complexity of improving health and wellbeing and undertaking public health work.

GOING FURTHER

Handy, C (1993) *Understanding Organisations* (4th edn). London: Penguin.
This is essential reading for anyone interested in organisations, by an eminent and influential writer on organisations who has been contributing to the development of organisational theory for more than three decades. This edition covers key concepts of motivation, leadership, power, role-playing and group-working culture, and questions of power and influence.

Mullins, LJ (2010) *Management and Organisational Behaviour* (9th edn). Harlow: Prentice-Hall.
This is a classic book on management and organisational theory, and very accessible. This edition contains clear and practical examples and case studies that provide a contemporary look at organisations. Areas covered include the organisational setting, the nature and context of organisations, organisational conflict, organisational structure and design and organisational culture, as well as many other engaging areas.

Pugh, DS and Hickson, DJ (2007) *Writers on Organizations* (6th edn). Harmondsworth: Penguin.
In this updated version of the 1964 book, the authors summarise the principal ideas on organisations, providing a comprehensive resource and overview of theory and practice in relation to organisations. The book covers organisational structure, local, national and international environments, the management of organisations, organisational decision-making and influence, people management and organisational change and learning.

Salaman, G (ed.) (2001) *Understanding Business Organisations*. London: Routledge.
Organisational theory is vitally relevant to today's student of business. This book introduces the student to classic debates and new perspectives on organisations through a wide-ranging but approachable selection of readings.

chapter 4

Leading Strategic Partnerships
Steve Whiteman and Vicki Taylor

Meeting the Public Health Competences

This chapter will help you to evidence the following competences for public health (Public Health Skills and Career Framework):

- Level 5(a) Knowledge of the principles of collaborative working and their application;
- Level 6(b) Knowledge of the principles and methods of partnership working and the benefits which collaboration can bring to the health and wellbeing of the population;
- Level 6(2) Identify opportunities and develop structures to take forward approaches to improve population health and wellbeing, including making use of partnership working;
- Level 7(2) Engage and influence others in and beyond own organisation to improve population health and wellbeing;
- Level 7(7) Review the effectiveness of collaborative working and make the necessary improvements;
- Level 7(a) Understanding of the principles and methods of partnership working and the benefits which collaboration can bring;
- Level 8(6) Review collaborative working and put in place the necessary improvements;
- Level 8(c) Understanding of the roles that various organisations, agencies, individuals and professionals play and the influences they may have on health and health inequalities;
- Level 8(d) Understanding of the principles of influencing, negotiating, facilitating and managing in a multi-agency environment to bring about change.

This chapter will also assist you in demonstrating the following National Occupational Standards for public health:

- Develop, sustain and evaluate joint work between agencies (SfJ_AD2);
- Map the environment in which your organisation operates (M&L_B2);
- Develop productive working relationships with colleagues and stakeholders (M&L_D2);
- Develop and sustain cross-sectoral collaborative working for health and wellbeing (PHS09).

In addition, this chapter will be useful in demonstrating Standards 9 and 11 of the Public Health Practitioner Standards:

Standard 9. Work collaboratively to plan and/or deliver programmes to improve health and wellbeing outcomes for populations/communities/groups/families/individuals.

Standard 11. Work collaboratively with people from teams and agencies other than one's own to improve health and wellbeing outcomes – demonstrating:

a. awareness of personal impact on others;
b. constructive relationships with a range of people who contribute to population health and wellbeing;
c. awareness of:

    i. principles of effective partnership working;
    ii. the ways in which organisations, teams and individuals work together to improve health and wellbeing outcomes;
    iii. the different forms that teams might take.

Overview

This chapter will help you to understand the potential benefits of partnership working for population health and wellbeing. It will assist you to develop your knowledge base in relation to:

- the benefits and costs to organisations of working across organisational boundaries;
- the range of practical and behavioural issues that need to be identified and addressed to make partnerships effective;
- how individuals within partnerships behave as negotiators, facilitators and leaders.

Changing population health behaviours to improve health outcomes and reduce health inequalities is a complex process. For public health professionals to be effective in addressing multi-factorial public health challenges such as obesity and alcohol misuse, they need to harness the full contribution of all stakeholders with a potentially beneficial role to play. In order to achieve this objective, public health professionals need to be able to identify, engage and work effectively with these stakeholders through mutual agreements and in multi-agency strategic partnerships.

The activities in this chapter will focus on:

- understanding why partnerships are seen as so critical to success in improving public health;
- exploring the role of public health professionals in partnership working;
- developing an understanding of the complexity of public health initiatives and the role of partnerships in addressing public health priority areas;
- appreciating the characteristics of highly-performing, effective partnerships;
- using an analytical framework to assess the effectiveness of a strategic partnership;
- exploring and understanding the roles that partnership members play, and considering the skills required to maximise the effectiveness of these roles.

This chapter uses theory, tools and case studies to explore partnerships for health. After reading this chapter you will be able to:

- identify the rationale for the importance of strategic partnerships in improving health and tackling health inequalities;

- describe the characteristics of effective partnerships (and of ineffective partnerships);

- articulate the roles that individuals within partnerships can play to make them effective in achieving organisational and shared goals.

Why strategic partnerships for health?

Public health objectives to improve health outcomes have a major focus on reducing risk factors for preventable conditions such as cardiovascular diseases, cancers, mental health disorders and sexually-transmitted infections within given populations. Such risk factors include a range of health behaviours (the 'causes' of preventable ill-health) and the underlying determinants of health (the 'causes of the causes').

Table 4.1 Risk factors

Examples of health behaviour risk factors (causes of preventable ill-health)	
Smoking	Poor diet
Low levels of physical activity	Obesity
Mental and emotional stressors	Drug and alcohol misuse
Risky sexual behaviour	Sunbathing and sunbed usage
Examples of determinants of health risk factors (causes of the causes)	
Poverty	Poor housing (cold, damp, overcrowded)
Worklessness	Violence in relationships
Fuel poverty	Crime and fear of crime
Quality of educational opportunities	Access to high-quality health services

Successive government strategies have identified that tackling these risk factors is key to improving public health and reducing health inequalities. These government strategies also have emphasised the central importance of multi-agency strategic partnership approaches to addressing these issues effectively.

Examples of recent government policies that accord priority to partnerships

In 2004, the government White Paper on public health, *Choosing Health: Making Healthier Choices Easier* (Department of Health, 2004a) emphasised that success would be based on partnerships and sharing information.

In 2006, the government White Paper on community services, *Our Health, Our Care, Our Say* (Department of Health, 2006b) reinforced the drive for a greater focus on improved health and wellbeing as a partnership between people and public services. Also in 2006, the government report *Health Challenge England: Next Steps for Choosing Health* (Department of Health, 2006a) stressed that action to improve health and care services will be underpinned through working in partnerships – between individuals, communities, business, voluntary organisations, public services and government.

In 2010, the coalition government White Paper on health, *Equity and Excellence: Liberating the NHS* (Department of Health, 2010a), made reference to the importance of partnership approaches, stating that:

> [W]e will simplify and extend the use of powers that enable joint working between the NHS and local authorities [...] local authorities' new functions will help unlock efficiencies across the NHS, social care and public health through stronger joint working.
>
> (Department of Health, 2010a, p34, p45)

The 2010 public health White Paper, *Healthy Lives, Healthy People* (Department of Health, 2010b), embraces strongly the importance of strategic partnerships to improve health and wellbeing:

> *Strong partnerships between communities, business and the voluntary sector will help address a range of health challenges.*
>
> (2010b, p48)

> *Directors of Public Health will be the strategic leaders for public health and health inequalities in local communities, working in partnership with the local NHS and across the public, private and voluntary sectors. The Government will shortly publish a response to the recent consultation on proposed new local statutory health and wellbeing boards to support collaboration across NHS and local authorities to meet communities' needs as effectively as possible.*
>
> (2010b, p51)

ACTIVITY 4.1

Think of a public health initiative you know well.

What partnerships were involved in this programme?

What is the advantage of a partnership approach?

Spend a few minutes thinking about these questions and jot down your thoughts.

Why are partnerships seen as so critical to success in improving public health?

> **Comment**
>
> At the most basic level, the answer is that no single agency or group working alone has the ability within its power or scope of influence to comprehensively address any one of these risk factors. Each risk factor is the product of a complex inter-play of cultural, social and economic influences and pressures on individuals and communities.

For example, whether a person smokes or not may seem to be a relative black and white issue on the face of it: one is either a non-smoker, or one exercises the choice to smoke. However, the factors that influence people to start smoking in the first place (usually, but not always, when they are young), or that lead to ex-smokers becoming smokers again, or that influence people to try but fail, or to try and suc-ceed in quitting smoking, are varied and complex. They are also different for differ-ent people. The box below sets out some of the factors that can influence individuals' smoking status.

Factors affecting individuals' smoking status

- Age;
- Family, cultural, ethnic and socio-economic background;
- How long a person has smoked for and how heavily they smoke
- Access to education about the health effects of smoking and the 'business' of the tobacco industry;
- The wider environments in which people live and work. These are important in determining their attitudes towards smoking and their intentions regarding con-tinuing to smoke or to quit. For example:
  - o the prevailing attitudes towards smoking in their family, social and work cir-cles (including workplace smoking policies);
  - o government policy regarding smoke-free environments and taxation related to tobacco products;
  - o the accessibility and availability of high-quality stop smoking support services;
  - o the effectiveness of public health media and social marketing campaigns designed to motivate people to quit smoking, through TV, radio, printed media, the internet, etc.

Let's look at another example in greater detail. Smoking has been the biggest public health challenge in the UK and in most western societies for decades. Many argue that obesity is now the biggest public health challenge for western societies, as we look forward to the decades ahead.

On a biological level, in the majority of cases, obesity is the result of a long-term imbalance between energy entering the body (through the food and drink that an individual consumes), and energy leaving the body (through core metabolic processes and the expenditure of energy through the movements of daily life – walking, running, housework, cycling, gardening, climbing stairs, etc.). Therefore, obesity results when *energy-in* exceeds *energy-out* over a protracted period of time.

It follows that the underlying determinants of obesity are chiefly those factors that influence what we consume and how physically active we are. This is easy to say, but start to list those determinants and it soon becomes apparent that they represent a highly complex, interconnected network of factors that operate at a range of levels.

ACTIVITY 4.2

Pause for a moment and think about obesity.

Can you list all those factors that that might influence the levels of obesity in the population?

Comment

It is likely that you identified a wide range of factors influencing the levels of obesity. Dahlgren and Whitehead (1991) developed a model that describes the main determinants of health across four layers: age, gender and genetic constitution are at the centre. Inevitably, these will influence people's health potential, but are fixed. The second layer is related to individual lifestyle factors and ways of living that have the potential to promote or damage health. The third layer is social and community influences and networks. These can provide mutual support for members of the community, but can also provide no support or have a negative effect. The fourth layer focuses on general socio-economic, cultural and environmental influences. These include structural factors such as housing, working conditions, agriculture and food production, access to services and provision of essential facilities.

Applying this model to obesity, the following level of detail and complexity emerges.

Given the range of complex factors that influence our eating behaviour and physical activity levels, it is apparent that there are a wide range of agencies and groups which have the potential to play a role in addressing aspects of these influences. As illustrated above, these organisations include the NHS and health service providers, local authority services, community organisations and groups, commercial organisations, policymakers and planners, individuals and communities themselves. If a strategy to tackle a complex issue such as obesity is to be addressed effectively, a co-ordinated approach involving all of the key stakeholders and interested parties needs to be brought together. This might be achieved, for example, by a high-level strategic partnership involving the core agencies overseeing the strategy, and a series of sub-groups focusing on specific areas of the strategy (commissioning weight management programmes, children and young people, older adults, etc.), bringing together operational managers and a wider range of agencies. If any significant stakeholders are missing from the table, then key pieces of the jigsaw are missing and the strategy will be more limited in what it can achieve.

Table 4.2 Analysis of influences on obesity (using the Dahlgren and Whitehead, 1991 model)

Four layers of determinants on health	*Some examples of the relationship with determinants of obesity*	*Examples of partner organisations and groups who could be well placed to address these influences*
Age, gender and hereditary factors	• Predisposition to obesity can be hereditary, so some people are at increased risk. Genetic factors can affect appetite, the rate at which you burn energy (metabolic rate) and how the body stores fat. However, even if your genes make weight gain more likely, it is not inevitable that you will be overweight. It is lifestyle that determines how the genes develop and that ultimately manages our weight • Studies have shown that the risk of obesity increases with age. For example, in 2006, about 34% of men and 32% of women aged 16 to 24 were overweight or obese, compared to 80% of men aged 55 to 64 and 73% of women aged 65 to 74 • Examples of genetic diseases linked to obesity are polycystic ovary syndrome (PCOS) and hypothyroidism • Medicines such as antidepressants, corticosteroids and oral contraceptives can cause weight gain	• Clinicians working with people with genetic disorders or taking medicines that contribute to weight gain are well placed to advise on lifestyle measures to help people to manage their weight • Patients can be referred to exercise on prescription classes and dieticians, for example
Individual lifestyle factors	• The choices we make as individuals regarding our diet and physical activity are the major factors determining whether we have a healthy weight. However, the environment into which we are born, live and age, the cultural values and beliefs that surround us and the commercial and political interests of our policymakers and business leaders all have an important influence on our ability to exercise free choice over our health behaviours • Babies and infants do not decide what they consume, the adults who feed them do • Breastfeeding protects against infant obesity, so babies who are exclusively breastfed have a lower risk of obesity than those who are bottle or mixed-fed	• Acute hospitals (midwives and doctors) • Health visitors and GP • Local authority • Children's Centres • Community centres and community support groups (such as breastfeeding advocate schemes) • School-based educational programmes

	• More than 10% of children starting their school career (in Reception year at age 4–5) are obese • The cost of and access to physical activity, healthy eating and weight management programmes • People's knowledge of how to eat healthily and exercise appropriately is variable. Walking is free and can be as beneficial to weight management and good health as paying to be a gym member	• Voluntary organisations • The availability of high-quality weight management programmes
Social and community networks	• The influence of family and friends on food choices and levels of physical activity • The availability of groups and networks that support physical activity and good diet, such as walking groups, cookery clubs, community breastfeeding support groups	• Self-help groups • Healthy eating community initiatives, such as cookery clubs and 'healthy shopping' schemes • Local physical activity schemes • Friends, family and community members
General socio-economic, cultural and environmental conditions	• Ability to access and afford healthy food in the locality • The availability of safe areas for children to play and adults to be physically active (such as parks) • The availability of safe and attractive travel options to support people to walk and cycle • Planning and development processes that take account of the need to design public environments which promote walking, cycling and safe play, enable access to affordable healthy food, and restrict obesogenic agents such as fast food outlets near schools • The availability of NHS (or affordable) local weight management groups for children and adults	• National and local government policy and legislation • National, regional and local lobby and campaigning, and expert organisations (e.g. National Obesity Forum and British Heart Foundation)

ACTIVITY 4.3

Within a strategic partnership to tackle obesity, what might the role of the public health specialist involve?

Think of the key activities you would expect public health to undertake.

Comment

You might have suggested some or all of the following roles:

- assessing the evidence base to capture a robust understanding of the factors that contribute to population obesity levels, and the interventions and programmes that can tackle these factors;
- conducting a stakeholder mapping exercise to identify who the key players are that need to be engaged in developing and implementing the strategy;
- facilitating the coming-together of the multi-agency partnership, and ensuring that strong organisational and leadership support are in place;
- working with all stakeholders to co-ordinate the process of developing and writing the strategy, ensuring that the aims and priorities of the strategy are clear and that local needs assessment is undertaken to inform prioritisation;
- working with stakeholders to design and put in place mechanisms to support the implementation, monitoring and evaluation of the strategy.

ACTIVITY 4.4

Choose a different public health priority, such as alcohol misuse or smoking, and undertake an analysis using the framework (see Table 4.3).

What does this analysis tell you about the range of partners with a role to play in addressing this public health priority area, and the complexity of the task?

Table 4.3 Framework for analysis of influences

Category of determinants on health	Some examples of the relationship with determinants of chosen public health priority area (e.g. smoking, alcohol misuse, etc.)	Examples of organisations and groups who could be well placed to address these influences
Age, gender and hereditary factors		
Individual lifestyle factors		
Social and community networks		
General socio-economic, cultural and environmental conditions		

Comment

If you selected smoking as your example, you may have noted that there is some evidence that people have different levels of addictiveness to nicotine linked to their genes *(hereditary factor)*.

Whether or not a person takes up smoking, although influenced by a wide range of factors, is essentially a modifiable individual health behavioural *(lifestyle factors)*.

Alcohol consumption can be strongly influenced by social and cultural factors, such as the behaviour of family and peers and social norms *(social and community factors)*. The cost of alcohol relative to a person's income (affected by taxation and potentially minimum pricing for alcohol), and legislation such as minimum age for purchasing alcohol and licensing laws, can all influence drinking behaviour *(socio-economic and environmental factors)*.

What's the evidence?

The National Institute for Health and Clinical Excellence (NICE) has published a range of evidence-based guidelines to support those responsible for planning or implementing strategies to improve public health and reduce health inequalities. These guidelines set out the different roles that key partners need to play in order to enable strategies to be effective. They include, for example, guidelines for reducing the prevalence of smoking within populations, increasing levels of physical activity among individuals and communities, and improving mental, social and emotional wellbeing among different groups. The fact that NICE has identified the need to provide a range of guidance for each public health topic area rather than a single guidance document, is in itself an indication of the complexity of the strategies that need to be implemented in order to be effective in addressing these public health priorities, and of the breadth of the partnerships required to implement them.

In its overarching guidance on behaviour change (NICE, 2007), the importance of taking multi-level approaches to enabling effective individual and population-level behaviour change to take place is identified. The guidance is intended to *provide a focus for children's trusts, health and wellbeing partnerships and other multi-sector partnerships working on health within a local strategic partnership* (NICE, 2007, p28) and recommends that robust plans need to be developed *in partnership with individuals, communities, organisations and populations to plan interventions and programmes to change health-related behaviour* (2007, p20).

There is overwhelming evidence that effective strategies for changing people's health-related behaviour can have a major impact on some of the largest causes of mortality and morbidity. The Wanless Report (2004) outlined a position in the future in which levels of public engagement with health are high, and the use of preventive and primary care services are optimised, helping people to stay healthy as they age.

The Wanless Report described the concept of the 'fully engaged' scenario as the best option for the future organisation and delivery of NHS services. This scenario involves a vision of changes in behaviours, with their social, economic and environmental context being at the heart of all disease prevention strategies. Such a future scenario cannot come about by chance; rather, only as the result of co-ordinated implementation of policy at national, regional and local levels, involving partnerships between public, private, third sector bodies and organisations, individuals and communities themselves.

Why do partnerships succeed or fail?

Partnerships essentially comprise people representing different interest groups, organisations or sometimes just themselves as members of local communities. They bring different interests, knowledge, insights, experience, resources and skills to the partnership agenda. Indeed, it is when action to address a public health priority requires this mix of skills, resources and qualities from different sectors and agencies that a partnership approach is needed. The most effective partnership identifies what the ingredients are that will be needed to develop an effective strategy, brings together the range of partners who collectively own these ingredients, and then works efficiently to harness the full impact of the partnership on public health outcomes.

ACTIVITY 4.5

What do you think are the characteristics of highly-performing, effective partnerships?

List as many characteristics as you can.

Comment

The Employers Organisation for Local Government describes a simple model for 'smarter partnerships', which includes four domains:

- leadership – partners share a vision and harness their energies to achieve more than they could on their own;
- trust – partners are mutually accountable, share risks and rewards fairly and support each other;
- learning – partners continuously seek to improve what they do in partnership;
- managing for performance – partners put in place the necessary practices and resources and manage change effectively.

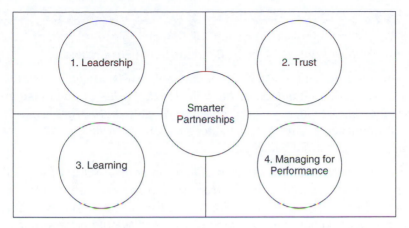

Figure 4.1 Smarter partnerships

Each domain within this model is necessary for the partnership to thrive. If any of these characteristics are absent or weak, the partnership will not perform effectively. The theory of effective partnerships is straightforward and logical to comprehend, but in practice there are often significant challenges and barriers that need to be addressed to ensure that the theory is put into practice effectively.

What's the evidence?

The Health Development Agency (which became part of NICE in 2005) identified a growing body of evidence (Audit Commission, 1998; Geddes, 1998; Pratt *et al.*, 1998; Employers Organisation for Local Government, nd) from inter-agency and collaborative practice which had led to an improved understanding of the factors that make partnerships effective. Their analysis of effective partnership working showed that these factors were centred on the following elements:

Leadership and vision – *the management and development of a shared, realistic vision for the partnership's work through the creation of common goals. Effective leadership is demonstrated by influencing, communicating with and motivating others, so that responsibility for decision-making is shared between partners.*

Organisation and involvement – *the participation of all key local players, and particularly the involvement of communities as equal partners. Not everyone can make the same contribution. Most voluntary organisations are small and locally based, with few staff. They may need resources and time to enable them to become fully engaged.*

Strategy development and coordination – *the development of a clear, community focused strategy covering the full range of issues supported by relevant policies, plans, objectives, targets, delivery mechanisms and processes.*

Development of local priorities for action will rely on the assessment of local needs, sharing of data, and a continuing dialogue between partners.

Learning and development – *effective partnerships will not only invest in shared objectives and joint outcomes, but will also add value through second-ments and other opportunities to share learning and contribute to professional and organisational development in partner organisations. Willingness to listen and to learn from each other builds trust.*

Resources – *the contribution and shared utilisation of information, financial, human and technical resources. The new freedoms to pool budgets and to pro-vide integrated services, for example between NHS primary care and local authority services, can help remove some of the traditional barriers to joint working. Cooperation can start by resourcing what everyone wants, for exam-ple, IT skills training.*

Evaluation and review – *assessing the quality of the partnership process and measuring progress towards meeting objectives. Partnerships need to demon-strate that they are making a difference and that meetings are more than talk-ing shops. They must also be able to show that they are making real improve-ments to services.*

Markwell *et al.* (2003, p5)

The following case study is an example of a partnership in practice, which dem-onstrates some of the strengths identified in the model of effective partnerships, and some of the challenges.

ACTIVITY 4.6

Read the following case study – Tobacco Control Partnership – and look at Table 4.4. Using this framework, assess the effectiveness of the Tobacco Control Partnership, and identify your ideas for how the partnership could be strengthened.

Case study	*Tobacco Control Partnership*
Background	The Tobacco Control Partnership has existed for three years in Area X. It was launched jointly by the chief executives of the borough council and the local NHS commissioning body at a full-day conference and launch event, which was attended by more than 150 people from a wide range of local organisations and communities. The minister for public health was invited to deliver the keynote speech at the launch event. The partnership was chaired initially by the director of public health, and is now chaired by the health improvement tobacco control lead. It meets four times a year.

Purpose	1. To jointly plan a range of actions to reduce smoking prevalence within Area X.
	2. To advise the council and local NHS commissioners on the effective deployment of resources to tackle the harm to public health caused by tobacco use.

Partners involved
: Middle managers from a number of council departments and NHS commissioners comprise the majority of regular attendees. These include environmental health, trading standards, children's services and public health. The voluntary sector is represented by the local voluntary sector co-ordinating organisation. Currently the private sector is not represented on the group.

Examples of work to date
: • The partnership has provided a network for the exchange of intelligence about tobacco control, smoking and health. Members of the group have visited other areas that have won awards for their tobacco control work, in order to learn from their success.

  • Social marketing insights work has been commissioned which has resulted in the implementation of a new awareness-raising campaign targeted at those sections of the local population which, local joint needs assessment show, have the highest rates of smoking.

  • There has been a steady increase in the numbers of people quitting smoking with the local stop smoking service over the last three years, including among the groups at greatest need.

  • School nurses have been trained to provide stop smoking services in schools. Uptake of this service to date has been low.

  • The partnership has not developed a documented strategy, but has preferred to focus on taking a small number of discrete projects forward.

  • A performance management framework has been discussed as a means to evaluate the effectiveness of the work. However, the person who was taking a lead on this work left 18 months ago, and it has not been progressed further.

Some issues
: • The partnership is accountable to the high-level health and well-being board for the area. In practice, this means that the board monitors progress according to the performance of the stop smoking service, and is generally assured that the partnership is working, as the stop smoking service figures are exceeding their targets.

  • The membership of the partnership has contracted in size – it used to be more extensive than now; a number of key players have begun to send apologies for absence on a regular basis. Private sector representatives have stopped attending.

  • A small number of people form the core group – they are all passionately committed to tobacco control work, but have a slightly different take on what the priorities should be. Two of the core group members in particular have had a number of disagreements in partnership meetings about what the group should be focused on, which has at times caused tensions and an uncomfortable atmosphere.

  • Originally, the group had been allocated a budget to support the project work (funded 50:50 from the council and the NHS). However, due to financial pressures elsewhere in the system, one party took a decision to remove their funding. The other party then reduced theirs to a minimal level.

- The chair of the group has proposed an 'away day' for the partnership. She wants the group to take time out to reassess its priorities, ways of working and its membership. She has proposed a facilitator to assist with this away day. The group were sympathetic to her suggestion at the last meeting, and agreed to go back to check with their managers if the time and resources required for such an event would be supported.

Table 4.4 Framework for analysing partnership effectiveness

Questions in key areas	Comment on the effectiveness of the partnership in this area	Suggestions for strengthening the partnership in these areas
Leadership and vision: does the partnership appear to have common agreed goals, shared targets, commitment and effort?		
Organisation and involvement: does there appear to be good participation of key stakeholders, agreement of relative roles, clarity of expectation? Are the right people at the right level involved?		
Strategy development and co-ordination: is there evidence of needs assessment and appropriate policies, plans, objectives, targets, delivery mechanisms, and funding?		
Learning and development: is there evidence of the partnership enabling the sharing of knowledge and skills across boundaries and groups and supporting innovation?		
Resources: is there evidence of the sharing of human, financial, technical and information resources?		
Evaluation and review: is the partnership clear about what success looks like, and whether it is achieving its goals?		

A systematic review of the role of partnerships in public health undertaken in 2008 by the School of Medicine and Health at Durham University in concluded that:

The majority of the literature on partnerships in public health focused upon partnership structures and processes and not outcomes.

Constantly changing policy priorities and organisational restructuring could have a detrimental impact on partnerships through having to re-negotiate the partnership with new or reconfigured agencies, or partnerships suddenly finding themselves faced with a new policy framework.

Area based partnership initiatives did not achieve better improvements to population health in contrast to comparator areas. However, there was some evidence that

partnership working had helped broaden organisational understanding of the wider determinants of health and/or push the issue of health inequalities up some organisations' agendas.

Not having the key personnel with authority to act on behalf of their respective organisations in a partnership was seen as a key deficit in successful partnership working.

'Local champions' were seen as crucial in partnerships to drive the policy agenda forward.

Partnerships suffered from not having the capacity to fulfil their policy priorities due to the lack of appropriate, or adequate, financial and human resources.

In some partnerships, many of the targets focused on partnership processes or activities rather than on health outcomes.

Smith *et al.* (2008, pp210–21)

What different roles do individuals play within partnerships?

As we have already seen in this chapter, strategic partnerships for health rely on the co-operation and effective joint working of agencies, communities and individuals to achieve shared goals and address shared priorities in order to improve health and tackle health inequalities. The individual partners typically send one or more representatives to partnership meetings, and allocate a proportion of their time to undertake work agreed at the partnership table.

ACTIVITY 4.7

Think of a partnership you know well.

Why were the different members of the partnership there?

What different roles did the members of the partnership take on?

Comment

The following are some examples of the reasons why individual members might be there.

- They have insights or expertise that is helpful to the various elements of the business of the partnership – this might include clinical expertise, experience of service delivery in a key area, expertise in literature review and assessing the evidence base in a given area, expertise in epidemiology, data analysis and interpretation, and insight into the needs of particular groups (for example, a community worker or resident from a given estate).
- The subject matter of the partnership is a key element of their job (e.g. one would expect a local teenage pregnancy co-ordinator to be a key player in the local teenage pregnancy partnership group).

- They might have a specific role as the commissioner of the services that are relevant to the partnership (e.g. in the case of the teenage pregnancy partnership, the commissioner of young people's sexual health services).
- They may be representing their organisation, taking a particular interest in a public health topic of critical importance to the organisation (for example, a director of children's services or a director of public health in an area of persistently high teenage conception rates may wish to chair the teenage pregnancy partnership).
- They may be there in a project support or administrative role, as effective partnerships need people whose job it is to make sure the business of the partnership is well organised, and that decisions are documented.

Whatever the reason for an individual being identified as appropriate to be a member of the strategic partnership, when they are engaging in the partnership's work, they need to have the skills to be able to operate in a number of different ways. Table 4.5 below provides a summary of some of the roles that are commonly used within partnership business, along with an analysis of why they are needed within this context, and some examples of when they are likely to be used effectively or ineffectively.

ACTIVITY 4.8

Think about a partnership in which you have been personally involved. Complete the following exercise to identify the roles you have played. Reflect on the skills you brought to bear when operating within these roles, and any development needs you may have in relation to the skills needed to be effective in the different roles.

Name of Partnership:
What was its main objective?

Role	Did you operate in this role? (Describe what you did.)	How confident and effective were you in this role?*	Do you have any learning needs to enable you to be more effective in this role in future?
Influencer			
Negotiator			
Facilitator			
Manager/organiser			
Leader			

* (Refer to the characteristics outlined in Table 4.5 below.)

Table 4.5 Roles that partnership members play

Partnership role	Why this role within partnerships?	Characteristics of effective qualities and behaviour in this role	Characteristics of ineffective qualities and behaviour in this role
Influencer	In the context of strategic partnerships for health, the ability to be influential is critical. This is because individuals within partnerships often have no direct authority over the other members of the group. Members are drawn from different agencies or groups, with their own management and governance arrangements, or may be community members. Often, no one member of the partnership (including the chair) can direct or instruct the others in a particular course of action. Actions need to be discussed, negotiated and agreed. In order to ensure that a desired approach is followed, an individual within a partnership needs to be influential.	An influential group member is likely to: • take time to understand the organisational priorities, cultures and targets of other partnership members; • provide credible evidence to the partners in a clear and accessible format to back up proposals; • have effective interpersonal and communication skills, such as strong listening, verbal and written skills; • be clear about the particular contribution that they are able to bring to the partnership, and be willing to share their resources, knowledge and experience accordingly; • be trusted and highly thought of by the group; • demonstrate authenticity in their commitment to the shared vision and goals of the partnership.	A less influential group member is likely to: • push their own agenda without considering the needs of the other partners; • use competitive behaviour, such as aggression rather than assertiveness; • attempt to blind other partners with jargon; • use their professional status or seniority to override or undermine other partners' contributions; • have poor listening and communication skills; • be unwilling to share resources, knowledge and experience; • lack personal credibility within the partnership.
Negotiator	Often within partnerships, negotiation is needed when a shared goal has been agreed, but there are differences of opinion about the best means of achieving that goal. It	An effective negotiator within a partnership is likely to: • be clear about the objective they are seeking to achieve, and have specific proposals to put on the table;	An ineffective negotiator within a partnership is likely to: • not have clear objectives or a planned approach to the negotiation process; • have failed to consider the needs and

	also can be required when resources are being allocated, or when partners are negotiating their respective roles in taking forward agreed actions. Multi-agency groups do not have the same hierarchy as usually exists within an individual organisation, and therefore agreements frequently need to be brokered, as they cannot simply be imposed from the top.	• have a planned approach to the negotiation process, involving a thought-out strategy; • have considered carefully the needs and aspirations of the other partners to the negotiation process; • be explicit with the other partners that they are entering into a negotiation process; • seek genuine win-win solutions to meet the needs of the other partners as well as their own; • be clear about 'deal breakers' – what would be an unsatisfactory outcome to the negotiation; • use assertive behaviour in seeking to achieve mutually acceptable solutions.	aspirations of the other parties to the negotiation; • be aggressive in the negotiation, seeking to achieve their own objective at all costs, or too passive, submitting to the proposals of others to avoid conflict situations and failing to achieve their own objectives; • fail to recognise when there is a need for negotiation.
Facilitator	Effective partnerships do not happen without significant time and investment from the various partners involved. Partnerships often have a great diversity of membership, which is a main reason for their strength, but also brings challenges with it. For example, there are often different professional groups with their own jargon, which can hinder communication with others. There may be people drawn	An effective facilitator within a partnership is likely to: • undertake a stakeholder analysis to ensure a good understanding of the different needs, values and ambitions of the various partners in the group; • invest time and effort in facilitating a genuine shared vision for the partnership and clear objectives to drive its joint strategy – this might be in the partnership meetings themselves, or through organising specific events (such as	An ineffective facilitator within a partnership is likely to: • fail to take proper account of the different cultures, contexts and constraints of the partners; • fail to invest sufficient time and effort in ensuring that the partnership operates effectively, that a clear shared vision drives the work, and that the group members operate in an environment of mutual trust and respect;

from quite different levels from their organisations or departments, creating dynamics relating to relative experience and seniority. There may be community members or service user representatives who may be unaccustomed to formal meetings, etc. In order to ensure that the diversity of members of the partnership is productive and does not hinder progress, facilitative roles are needed. Within partnerships, the role of the chair is often facilitative rather than directive. A co-ordinator, such as a teenage pregnancy or obesity co-ordinator, is also often well placed to take a facilitative role in a partnership. Also senior public health specialists often need to adopt facilitator roles to be effective in their partnership working.

As this chapter has shown, strategic partnerships are often complex 'virtual' teams of people drawn from a wide range of different organisations and groups. In order to ensure that the business of the partnership is transacted effectively,

partnership development days) to ensure that sufficient protected time is given to building trust and vision across the partnership;

- ensure that opportunities are provided for the partnership to review how it is operating – for example, this can be achieved through the use of partnership assessment tools;
- have strong interpersonal and relationship management skills and abilities;
- be skilled in dealing with conflict and turning potentially destructive situations into constructive learning experiences.

- fail to facilitate regular partnership review activities;
- have poor interpersonal and communication skills, such as listening skills;
- avoid conflict situations or be unskilled in dealing with them when they arise.

Manager/organiser

Effective managers or organisers within a partnership context are likely to:

- be highly organised and skilled in generic business processes;
- have good interpersonal skills to enable effective communication with a range of people across organisational boundaries;

Ineffective managers or organisers within a partnership context are likely to:

- be disorganised and inexperienced in administrative work;
- have poor communication skills, and find it difficult to communicate with different groups of people;

	the partnership and its processes need to be well organised and managed. Meetings, agendas, reports and papers need to be organised in a timely and consistent manner. Communication systems between partners and wider interested parties (e.g. through newsletters or websites) need to be considered. Action plans need to be written, and their implementation monitored and documented. Data and intelligence need to be gathered, analysed and disseminated. Meetings need to be chaired and structured to ensure that the core business is covered. Effective partnerships require a lot of management.	• be a good planner, thinking ahead effectively, scheduling milestones within plans working backwards from key deadlines; • be flexible and adaptable, as partnerships can shift their focus and external factors (such as a change in government policy) can alter deadlines and change priorities with little notice; • be able to chair or facilitate meetings when required; • be effective at meeting deadlines and supporting others to complete their tasks within agreed timeframes.	• be inexperienced at long-term planning within a multi-agency context; • find the need to be flexible and adaptable a challenge; • not have chairing or facilitation experience; • struggle to meet deadlines and progress chase others to meet their deadlines.
Leader	With a wide range of different people often involved within a partnership for health, the need for strong leadership is critical. Leadership may come from the chair of the partnership, but also may be exhibited by any of the partnership members at different times within the process. For example, A public health or clinical expert could	Effective leaders within partnerships for health are likely to: • be excellent communicators, skilled at getting their message across and able to command and retain the attention of others; • have credibility across a range of players and agencies; • have clarity of thought and vision, able to retain what is most important to the	Ineffective leaders within partnerships for health are likely to: • have poor communication skills, failing to communicate their message clearly, losing their audience's attention; • lack credibility among the partnership members, failing to achieve trust and respect; • fail to retain a clear focus on the main purpose of the partnership work,

provide leadership in making a compelling case for the need for the partnership work, communicating effectively how many lives could be saved, or how quality of life could be improved though the work of the group. Leadership is needed to ensure that the group develops and maintains a strong sense of shared purpose, and remains highly motivated and committed to the partnership. Leadership is often required back within individual organisations, to advocate for resources to be allocated to the partnership's work and to ensure that the corporate prioritisation process takes account of the issue addressed by the partnership. In addition, leadership can be demonstrated through more background processes, such as using data and intelligence to illuminate important new local knowledge about a particular issue.

ambitions of the partnership at all times;

- have the skills to keep the partnership together, heading in the same direction when distractions or competing priorities threaten to derail the work.

becoming easily distracted by competing demands.

Chapter summary

This chapter has considered three specific aspects relating to strategic partnership for health across organisational boundaries:

1. Why strategic partnerships for health?
2. Why do partnerships succeed or fail?
3. What different roles do individuals play within partnerships?

Partnerships were considered to be essential for a number of reasons. Complex public health problems require complex solutions, and no one agency working alone has the ability to resolve this complexity. Effective partnerships provide a greater chance of improving things for local people through, for example, bringing about the sharing of intelligence, improving understanding of the needs and wants of a local community and facilitating the sharing of resources. Partnerships can bring about a greater degree of challenge and scrutiny than single agency working, especially when local people become involved, helping to deliver the best solution rather than the easiest solution to complex problems. Partnerships can be effective in identifying and addressing gaps and reducing unnecessary duplication of effort. They can bring about opportunities for shared learning across organisations, and support the development of good relationships which can have lasting benefits beyond the life of a specific initiative. Sometimes partnerships are needed when they are made a statutory requirement, or there is a strong policy expectation from central government: for example, partnerships to produce the Joint Strategic Needs Assessment; partnerships operating as the Local Safeguarding Children's Board; and Health and Wellbeing Partnerships.

Effective and successful partnerships require common agreed goals, shared targets, commitment and effort. They also require the participation of key stakeholders and agreement about roles. Needs assessment, clear policies and plans with clear delivery mechanisms and dedicated funding to support these activities are elements found in successful partnerships. Learning and development within partnerships, sharing resources, skills and knowledge and a clear vision of what constitutes success are all important to the success of partnership working.

A range of roles that are important in successful partnership working were identified. These included the roles of influencer, negotiator, facilitator, manager and leader.

GOING FURTHER

Department of Health (2000) *Working in Partnership: Developing a Whole Systems Approach*. London: HMSO.
  This document provides a good practice guide and contains some interesting examples of partnership working.

Gunn, LA (1978) Why is implementation so difficult? *Management Services in Government*, 33: 169–76.
A paper setting out Gunn's analysis of the 10 main challenges for the implementation of strategies to improve health at the local level, with a particular focus on health inequalities.

Hamer, L (2004) *Pooling Resources Across Sectors: A Report for Local Strategic Partnerships*. London: Health Development Agency.
A succinct and useful resource developed by the National Primary and Care Trust Development Programme, which sets out some key lessons on developing successful partnerships.

Health Development Agency (2005) *Tackling Health Inequalities: Learning from the East and West Midlands Partnerships*. Wetherby: Health Development Agency.
A succinct and useful resource developed by the National Primary and Care Trust Development Programme that sets out some key lessons on developing successful partnerships. Available to download at: **www.nice.org.uk/aboutnice/whoweare/ aboutthehda/hdapublications/hda_publications.jsp?o=550**

Leathard, A (1994) *Going Inter-Professional: Working Together for Health and Welfare*. London: Routledge.
This book provides a considered discussion of the case for working inter-professionally for health. A critical analysis of inter-professional working, a theoretical background to inter-professional work and practice issues in promoting health is debated. The inter-professional approach is sometimes seen as a threat to the identities and training of the individual professions involved. The contributors to this book draw on a range of considerable experience to confront these issues and point to positive ways forward. Chapters 6 and 8 are particularly pertinent.

Pratt, J, Gordon, P and Plampling, D (1998) *Partnership: Fit for Purpose*. London: The King's Fund.
This text offers a way of thinking about the purpose of partnership, considering different partnership behaviours that fit different purposes. Focusing on co-evaluation, the text describes an approach that can lead to sustainable solutions to local problems.

Plampling, D, Gordon, P and Pratt, J (2000) Practical partnerships for health and local authorities. *British Medical Journal* 320, 1723–5.
The last in a series of articles seeks to discuss the differing types of partnership that exist, and to promote the notion that all partnerships need to find a shared goal and build trust gradually. Some key lessons on effective partnership are set out.

chapter 5

Skills for Leading
Vicki Taylor

Meeting the Public Health Competences

This chapter will help you to evidence the following competences for public health (Public Health Skills and Career Framework):

- Level 5(2) Lead on discrete areas of work;
- Level 5(3) Identify and influence other people and agencies in own area of work to improve population health and wellbeing;
- Level 5(6) Communicate using various techniques appropriate to the audience and the purpose of the communication;
- Level 5(b) Knowledge of methods of effective communication;
- Level 6(f) Knowledge of negotiation and influencing approaches and skills and their application;
- Level 7(2) Engage and influence others in and beyond own organisation to improve population health and wellbeing;
- Level 7(5) Advocate for health and wellbeing and reducing health inequalities;
- Level 7(e) Understanding of the importance of negotiation and influencing skills and their application;
- Level 7(f) Knowledge of the basic management models and theories associated with motivation and leadership;
- Level 8(3) Improve the population's health and wellbeing through effective use of negotiating, influencing, facilitation and management skills within a multi-agency environment.

This chapter will also assist you in demonstrating the following National Occupational Standards for public health:

- Provide leadership for your team (M&L_B5);
- Provide leadership in your area of responsibility (M&L_B6);
- Develop and sustain effective working with staff from other agencies (SFJ AD1);
- Advocate for the improvement of health and wellbeing (PHP47);
- Represent one's own agency at other agencies' meetings (CJ_F408);
- Communicate effectively with the public and others about improving the health and wellbeing of the population (PHS11).

In addition, this chapter will be useful in demonstrating Standards 11 and 12 of the Public Health Practitioner Standards:

Standard 11. Work collaboratively with people from teams and agencies other than one's own to improve health and wellbeing outcomes – demonstrating:

a. awareness of personal impact on others;
b. constructive relationships with a range of people who contribute to population health and wellbeing.

Standard 12. Communicate effectively with a range of different people using different methods.

Overview

This chapter will help you to develop negotiation, persuasion and influencing skills and to consider the implications for leading public health and health improvement. Also, it will help you to develop your thinking about the nature of negotiation, persuasion and influence and how they differ from each other. Principled negotiation is offered as a strategy for creating more successful negotiation outcomes. Push, pull, persuasive, preparatory and preventative influence strategies are presented and their relevance for public health assessed. The nature of power and differing types of power are introduced. Theses include French and Raven's sources of power, namely, 'Reward power, Coercive power, Legitimate power, Referent power and Expert power'. Other models are considered, including the expert and positional power and persuasive influence proposed by Handy. Finally, we will consider the importance of understanding yourself and the communication process in order to maximise your effectiveness in promoting and securing health improvement.

The activities in this chapter will focus on:

- clarifying the differences between persuasion, influence and negotiation;
- understanding when and how to use persuasion, negotiation and influence;
- appreciating the strengths and weaknesses of different approaches to negotiation and influence, and their potential use in improving population health and wellbeing;
- understanding the importance of negotiation, persuasion and influencing skills;
- appreciating the significance of effective communication and the communication process.

This chapter uses theory, tools and case studies to explore the relationship between persuasion, influence and negotiation. The nature of power and the communication process are explored also, using theory, tools and case studies.

After reading this chapter you will be able to:

- articulate the difference between negotiation, influence and persuasion;
- appreciate the strengths and weaknesses of different approaches to influence, persuasion and negotiation;
- assess which influencing strategies you use most frequently;
- examine the ways in which you use power and aim to use power responsibly;
- articulate ideas about the communication process and identify effective ways of communicating for health improvement.

The relationship between influence, persuasion and negotiation

Public health operating across and within organisations is a challenging area of work. To be effective as a public health leader requires an ability to influence others and create changes that will lead to health improvements. Negotiation, influence and persuasion processes are critical for the delivery of public health and health improvement where working together to achieve health improvement requires agreeing on programmes, priorities and resource allocation and prioritisation. The need to influence which programmes are implemented and how, often across multi-agency partnerships, is central. This has gained increasing recognition in public health both in the UK and internationally, as the ability to negotiate and influence others is acknowledged as a core public health competence.

However, the role of negotiation and influence within the development of programmes to achieve health improvement is not always explicitly recognised. Until recently, and despite the importance of leadership and management skills, including influencing others, persuasion and negotiation, these skills have had less of a focus in comparison to the development of public health knowledge and skills such as critical appraisal. Looking at any of the models, frameworks and theories that focus on the development (and indeed planning) of public health programmes, there is little explicit reference to influencing others or negotiation skills.

Nutbeam and Wise comment on the importance of developing substantial skills in the behavioural, social and political sciences in order for the public health workforce to influence the structural and environmental determinants of health, in addition to influencing health behaviours (Nutbeam and Wise, 2002, p1883). In the chief medical officer's review of the public health function, it was concluded that public health requires a *facilitative, influencing style that can make use of horizontal networks in addition to vertical command and control networks* (Department of Health, 2001, p32). Influencing, persuading and negotiating with others are central to the public health role and achieving health improvement. In their consideration of evidence-based policy and practice (what they refer to as public health action), Rychetnik *et al.* (2004) stress the importance of advocacy and lobbying and influence in public health, and acknowledge that the *process of achieving influence is often more difficult, and requires more complex social and political negotiations, than appraising evidence and formulating recommendations* (2004, p541). Developing and building relationships, *based on influence rather than direction and control* (Dooris and Hunter, 2007, p117), are seen as the key to taking forward a multi-sectoral approach to a health agenda.

Working to improve public health requires you to influence people, put health improvement on the agenda and prioritise initiatives that can contribute to health improvement. More often than not, this is achieved through gaining support from others, by galvanising interest, influencing and inspiring others, sometimes involving persuasion and negotiation. Let's now explore these terms in more detail.

ACTIVITY 5.1

What do the terms *persuading*, *negotiating* and *influencing* mean to you?

Can you think of situations where you have used any (or each) of these?

What distinction would you make between negotiation, persuasion and influence?

Comment

Persuading involves being able to convince others to take a particular action: for example, working to get others to see that action to improve health should be a priority. From a public health perspective, persuasion is getting people to *want* to do what you want them to do, in order to achieve improvements in health. In a previous role as assistant director of public health I would have had no hesitation in admitting that I wanted the staff in the two London boroughs in which I worked to take on responsibility for health gain in local schools, for focusing on housing and considering how the built environment might be developed in order to enhance the health and wellbeing status of local residents and employees. Successfully persuading and then getting people to tell me that they were responsible for improving health and wellbeing were the greatest accolades I could have hoped for. Also, having the director of education telling me that the health improvements in young people were in her domain pleased me greatly. Persuasion was an important technique that I used to convince others that they had a role to play in improving the health and wellbeing of local residents and employees.

Negotiation

This involves a dialogue between two or more people or parties that is intended to reach an understanding – hopefully mutually agreed. It involves being able to discuss and agree a mutually satisfactory outcome, even though both parties may have differing views and opinions about what that might be. Successful negotiation is characterised by leaving both parties with a sense of win-win and finding the outcome acceptable. As such, negotiation is a two-way process and usually involves a common focus between the parties, although they may have differing perspectives about the desired outcome. Successful negotiation should result in both parties feeling positive about the outcome. Phases or stages in a negotiation are often referred to: these involve moving through each stage, where issues and potential disagreements can be worked through, and a successful outcome reached. Although differing stages are commonly referred to, there is general agreement that there are at least three phases: preparation, negotiation and closing (see Table 5.1).

Table 5.1 A typical rational model for negotiation

Stage	Explanation
Phase I: Planning	Prepare for the negotiation by understanding: 1. The facts 2. Assumptions 3. Customer needs 4. Negotiable components 5. Your own bottom-line concessions.

Phase II: Conducting the Negotiation	An open discussion to help 'set the stage' for the conduct of the negotiation. Options to consider are:
	1. General introductions and small-talk to establish rapport (reinforcement of the importance of 'win-win')
	2. Definition of the problem/concern and its impact
	3. Overview of the purpose, goals and objectives
	4. An open 'questioning' phase when both parties have the opportunity to:
	  a. Assess the needs and interests of the other parties (e.g. to test assumptions).
	  b. Discuss possibilities to gain mutual satisfaction (e.g., negotiable components).
	  c. Establish objective decision criteria/standards.
	  d. Identify ways to assist the other parties to negotiate within their organisation.

Phase III: Closing	1. Make concessions to reach agreement and mutual satisfaction 2. Ensure that agreement/satisfaction has been reached 3. Identify specific action plans to implement 4. End on a positive note.

Source: **www.richardchangassociates.com/pdfs/epins.pdf** (last accessed October 2011). Reproduced with kind permission.

Influencing

This includes both persuasion and negotiation. In influencing someone, the goal is to try to get the person to do something or to support you. For example, in trying to influence others to promote health, usually you are attempting to get them to provide support for health improvement; this in turn may mean changing their attitude and/or behaviour and, in some cases, their priorities. Influence is often a one-way process and may be direct and indirect in approach, but essentially it refers to one person (or a group) affecting what another person (or group) does or thinks. A variety of influencing strategies exist, ranging from those that try to 'pull' others along, to those that aim to persuade others.

What's the evidence?

Fisher *et al.* (1999, p7) maintain that negotiation traditionally involves a series of moves whereby participants successively take, and then give up a sequence of positions. This pattern of taking and giving up positions serves a useful purpose in that it makes transparent to both parties what each party is seeking. However, Fisher *et al.* argue that *'positional bargaining' fails to meet the basic requirements of a wise agreement, efficiently and amicably* (1999, p7). One of the fundamental flaws of positional bargaining is that it is rooted in 'win-lose' assumptions, whereby there are either irreconcilable positions or both parties inevitably compromise and accept a scarcely satisfactory outcome.

Fisher *et al.* (1999, p10) offer an alternative approach that they refer to as *principled negotiation*. They advocate four basic principles:

1. people – separate the people from the problem;
2. interest – focus on interests not positions;
3. options – generate a variety of possibilities before deciding what to do;
4. criteria – insist on objective criteria.

These principles or approaches to negotiation are central throughout the stages of negotiation.

ACTIVITY 5.2

Who do you need to negotiate with in order to improve health in your area of work?

How might you go about doing this?

What resources would you use?

What difficulties might you encounter, and how could you handle these?

How might the four principles suggested by Fisher *et al.* help?

Comment

Separating the people from the problem requires an approach that preserves social interaction and the relationships between parties. This enables attention to be focused on achieving a satisfactory outcome rather than on problems of perception, emotion or communication. Fisher *et al.* (1999) suggest strategies for managing problems of perception, defusing emotional problems in the negotiation process and techniques for minimising communication problems (summarised in Table 5.2). Three types of communication problems are identified:

1. not talking to one another;
2. not listening to one another; and
3. misunderstanding or misinterpreting each other.

As they note, without communication there can be no negotiation (Fisher *et al.*, 1999, p20).

Table 5.2 Strategies for managing 'people' problems in negotiations

Strategies for managing problems of perception

1. Attempt to see the situation from the other party's perspective. Try to understand what they think and feel, and why they think and feel as they do.
2. Avoid making assumptions and fearing the worst.
3. Avoid blaming the other party for the problem. Blame is generally counterproductive.
4. Discuss each other's perceptions. Such discussion may reveal shared perceptions, strengthen the parties' relationship and facilitate productive negotiations.
5. Seek opportunities to dispel misperceptions that the other party may have about you.
6. Give your opponent a stake in the outcome by making sure that they participate in the negotiation process.
7. Make your proposals consistent with the principles and self-image of the other party, so that they can reconcile the outcome with their principles and ensure that it does not compromise their integrity.

Strategies for defusing emotional problems

1. Recognise and understand emotions and try to understand them.
2. Make emotions explicit and acknowledge them as legitimate.
3. Allow the other party to 'let off steam'.
4. Avoid reacting to emotional outbursts.
5. Use symbolic gestures such as sympathy, a statement of regret or a shaking of hands.

Techniques for minimising communication problems

1. Listen actively and acknowledge what is being said – this involves paying close attention to what is said and repeating what you have heard.
2. Speak to be understood – try to put yourself in the other person's position and consider where they might see the situation differently.
3. Speak about yourself rather than the other person. This is an important technique and enables the conveying of a position without provoking a defensive reaction.
4. Speak for a purpose – especially as sometimes the communication problem is one of too much being said. Knowing what you want to communicate and the purpose that this information will serve will help the process.

Source: Adapted from Fisher *et al.* (1999)

Focusing on interests, not positions

This requires a focus on what the parties really want, rather than a negotiating position. This enables parties in the negotiation to identify common areas of interest and avoid focusing on a 'bottom line'. It also helps to focus attention on the problem rather than respective organisations and roles. Fisher *et al.* (1999) argue that focusing on interests enables them to generate options for mutual gain. Identifying and generating a range of possibilities can be likened to using a problem-solving technique which attempts to identify potential new solutions that will create the possibility for a win-win outcome. Using techniques such as 'brainstorming', which are designed to generate as many ideas as possible to solve the problem at hand, can be powerful. However, the key ground rule is to postpone all criticism and evaluation of ideas until the next stage. Identifying objective criteria for decisions is the fourth principle proposed by Fisher *et al.*, and where these can be found, they argue that the negotiation process can be simplified enormously.

Finally, Fisher *et al.* advise negotiators to know what their Best Alternatives to A Negotiated Agreement (BATNA) are, and advocate this especially when the other side is powerful. They stress that unless you are clear about this, there is the possibility of accepting an agreement that is far worse than the one you might have got, or of rejecting one that is far better than you might otherwise achieve.

ACTIVITY 5.3

Think about your current role and note all those situations in which you need to influence others.

What does influencing involve?

What aspects do you find easy about influencing people in these situations?

What aspects do you find difficult?

Comment

You might have identified the need to use different strategies in different contexts and with different people, and to adapt your approach to the context. You may have identified that you use particular strategies to influence people in your own organisation, and other strategies to influence those in partner organisations. For example, you might have given greater weight to an evidence-informed approach with those in partner organisations. (Activity 5.4 explores this in more detail.) Six different types of influence strategy are usually written about in the management literature, often collectively referred to as the 'Six Ps'. These include using *position* or *authority*, push and pull strategies, persuasion, preparatory and preventive strategies.

The 'Six Ps' influencing strategies

Position (or authority)

These may be used in order to influence others, and the success of this strategy will be dependent on how authority is exercised in an organisation. For most public health professionals who work across organisations and often lead without authority, this strategy is likely to have a number of drawbacks. For example, there may be ambiguity over how positional authority is defined, and different people in different organisations are likely to have conflicting and differing perspectives on what is legitimate.

Push strategies

These attempt to influence others by imposing 'sanctions' if the people concerned do not do what is required. In a context where partnerships and collaborative working are paramount, this does not seem to be a particularly useful influencing strategy to achieve public health and health improvement goals. The risk of such an approach is that there is reduced commitment and motivation, and a climate of mistrust and destructive conflict.

Pull strategies

These often draw on rewards (or exchanges of some sort) in order to influence others, and are dependent on the reward offered being valued. Expertise may be offered or support for another area of work that is valued by the other party, or may simply involve favour or inclusion in a group or working party on another area of public health that is valued. Pull strategies can be useful in public health, but care needs to be taken to ensure that such strategies are not perceived as unfair.

Persuasive strategies

These achieve influence by trying to change someone's attitude (or behaviour), to get them to want to do something or want to support you in some way. Because persuasion involves appealing to reason through argument, it is a popular and successful means of influence. Once persuaded, people will want to do what you want them to do. From a public health perspective this can be a very successful strategy. For example, in a previous public health role I recall providing a summary of a smoke alarm scheme in the USA which had mobilised community support and achieved a significant reduction in death rates from fires through the installation of smoke alarms in lower socio-economic housing. In discussing this scheme with the then director of environmental health, a dialogue in which we attempted to understand each other's viewpoint was instrumental in gaining support for a similar scheme to be established, and in securing some funding towards the programme.

Preparatory strategies

These involve building relationships with others who may need to be involved or influenced at some point in the future. Such strategies underpin the development of a wide range of partnerships for health improvement. Networking, coalition-building and developing strong relationships with key stakeholders are central to this approach.

Preventative strategies

These can be used to achieve influence, for example, by stopping questions being raised, suppressing opposition and dissent and retaining information. These activities can be deemed acceptable, as in the case of lobbying and advocacy, and are interlinked with interpersonal and political skills. Such strategies can be very effective in achieving public health goals; however, it is important to consider how acceptable such strategies may be with the many differing stakeholders involved in achieving health improvement.

ACTIVITY 5.4

Think about your own area of work. What authority, if any, does your position give you to influence the work of other people?

Have there been any occasions where you have tried to make use of push strategies to influence people's behaviour? Was this an effective strategy? If not, why?

Have you used pull strategies to influence others? Can you think of an occasion when someone tried to influence you using a pull or reward strategy? If so, how did it make you feel? What are the implications of using this approach in order to influence others?

Can you think of an occasion where you have used persuasion effectively in order to influence others? To what extent was it successful? What factors do you think contributed to it being successful?

Consider an occasion that was less successful. What factors do you think might have contributed to this?

Consider a public health initiative that you are currently working on. What support do you need in order to take this work forward? Who might you need to influence? What do you need to do in order to develop and maintain the support you need??

Can you identify occasions when preventative strategies were used? What was the outcome? How effective was this as an approach to influencing others? Can you see any potential strengths or weaknesses of this approach?

Comment

Push strategies, by their very nature, are only likely to be effective in situations where there is no real alternative, such as a crisis. They are unlikely to be useful in the context of working together with others to improve public health. However, there may be occasions where imposing a cost such as public criticism is justified (i.e. not working to improve health, actively undergoing processes that may reduce health and wellbeing outcomes). The main drawback of push strategies is that they can lead to a climate of fear and distrust.

Pull or reward strategies also have pros and cons. They can be used to influence others (for example, allowing a multinational food supplier to be actively included within a food and health partnership, provided that they agree to ensure that a greater number of 'healthier' foods are included in price reductions). While this may be effective in the short term, it is less clear how effective this approach is in the longer term.

Using persuasion based on genuine dialogue can be a very effective approach, although care needs to be taken to ensure that the boundary between persuasion and other strategies does not become blurred. Often, persuasion can be linked with pull or reward strategies.

Preparatory strategies attempt to prepare the ground for developing strong relationships with key stakeholders. However, one of the potential pitfalls is that sometimes stakeholders can perceive there to be manipulation. Developing coalitions and working to build genuine relationships can help to prevent this.

Preventative strategies can be very effective in achieving influence, provided that the methods used are deemed to be acceptable to those with whom you are working.

ACTIVITY 5.5

Think about a particular piece of work you are currently engaged in with others to improve health. Now consider the areas that you need to influence and ask yourself the following questions.

What exactly do I wish to achieve?

Which of my objectives must I achieve?

What other options are acceptable to me?

How might this fit with what others want?

What is my impact on others, and how might this make them feel?

Ideas about power

Power is a complex and important phenomenon for the public health workforce to understand. This is particularly important, given the political nature of health and wellbeing. Linstead *et al.* suggest that power is *one of the most enduring aspects of human relationships* (2004, p183). Northouse considered there to be two types kinds of power in organisations: position power and personal power. Position power is derived from the position that someone holds in the organisation, while personal power is derived from interaction and the relationship with *followers* (2001, p6). This view of power is closely related to working in an organisation and does not seem to have the same resonance when working on the boundary or margins of a number of different organisations, or being employed by more than one organisation, as is the case for many public health workers. French and Raven's (1959) consideration of power is similar, in that it views power from the perspective of those who are managed. They identified five sources of power:

1. reward power – this comes from the control of resources;

2. coercive power – this embodies the fear of punishment perceived by the staff member;

3. legitimate power – this is linked with the role or authority that someone has;

4. referent power – this comes from the personal characteristics or charisma that the manager has;

5. expert power – this is based on expertise.

French and Raven noted that the use of different types of power is dependent on the situation, and that managers used a range of types of power. Handy (1999[1976]) develops these ideas about power and separates out influence as another important dimension. He proposes that power is not a fixed concept, but rather one that is relational and a product of social interaction. The most common power resources are resource and position power, although expert and personal power are seen as becoming more important. From a public health perspective, personal and expert power and persuasive influence seem to be the most significant. Mintzberg (1983b) describes the political games commonly found in organisations (summarised in

Table 5.3, and described in more detail in Chapter 7). You might like to review each of these and identify those resources that you use.

Table 5.3 Power in and across organisations

Different models of power		
French and Raven (1959): Five forms of power	Reward, Coercive, Expert, Referent, Legitimate	
Handy (1999[1976]): Power resources and influence	*Power* Physical, resource, position, expert, negative, personal	*Influence* Force, rules, persuasion, ecology, magnetism
Mintzberg (1983b): Political games	*Categories* Games to resist authority, counter-resistance, to build power base, to change the organisation	Insurgency game, counter-insurgency game, sponsorship game, alliance-building game, empire-building game, budgeting game, expertise game, lording game, line manager vs. staff game, rival camps game, strategic candidates game, whistle-blowing game and 'Young Turks' game

Source: Adapted from French and Raven (1959), Handy (1999[1976]) and Mintzberg (1983b)

Effective negotiation and influencing requires clarity about what needs to be achieved and a good sense of available options. In addition to being well informed about the public health evidence and implications, your attributes as a public health leader (enthusiasm, energy, clarity of vision, flexibility, social and interpersonal skills) will play an important role in determining how effective you are. An understanding of yourself and the impact that you have on others is critical. How you influence others will reflect your own values and, in turn, how successful you are will be dependent on how those you are trying to influence perceive your influence strategies and how effectively you communicate with them. An ability to demonstrate empathy and to adapt to others and communicate in terms that can be understood is also important.

Communicating effectively

Effective communication is important in achieving health improvement, especially in the context of working across organisational boundaries and with many different organisations and partnerships. Furthermore, interpersonal relationships and communication form the basis for most aspects of partnership working and working within organisations. Mintzberg's (1971) study of managers demonstrated that they spend an average of 78 per cent of their time on verbal communication, thus reiterating the significance of communication.

Shannon and Weaver first developed a model of communication in 1949, which looked at how information was communicated from one person to another and how it was received. In this model even the simplest communication involves seven stages.

Stage 1: the sender wants to convey something to the receiver.

Stage 2: the message is encoded by the sender.

Stage 3: when the sender is satisfied with the encoding of the message, they transmit it.

Stage 4: the message transfers from the sender to the receiver.

Stage 5: the receiver decodes the message.

Stage 6: the receiver understands the idea that the sender wished to communicate.

Stage 7: the receiver takes action as a result of the message (Shannon and Weaver, 1949).

The communication process also can be illustrated as a cycle where the sender and receiver are in a continuous process of encoding, decoding, receiving and sending messages (Figure 5.1).

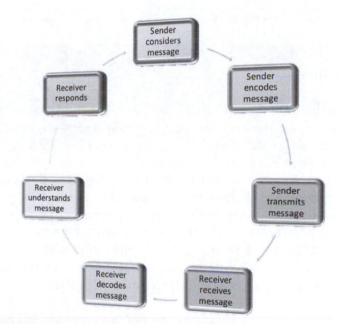

Figure 5.1 Communication process

ACTIVITY 5.6

Think about situations where you need to communicate.

How do you ensure that the message received is what you intended?

What actions do you take to ensure that you get feedback?

How do you ensure that 'noise' doesn't interfere with the message?

Look at each of the stages set out in Shannon and Weaver's very simple model and/or the stages set out in Figure 5.1.

How might you use these to make your communication more effective?

Comment

Interference (noise, distraction, misunderstanding, assumptions, cultural or value differences, etc.) can occur at any stage and for this reason, feedback and confirmation are essential. Shannon and Weaver suggest that 'noise' or interference serve to affect the message, so that the message received is not always the same as intended. Feedback processes enable the message sender to ensure that what is received was what was intended. There is often a big difference between what is transmitted and what is received; therefore, it is critical to ensure that what is received and what is transmitted are the same via a feedback loop. The communication process is complicated further by perception and the physical, social and cultural context (Buchanan and Hucyzinski, 2004).

Chapter summary

In this chapter we began by considering the relationship between influence, persuasion and negotiation. The need to influence, often across organisational boundaries, has been given greater attention than previously. However, despite this importance, it was acknowledged that developing these skills has been less of a priority in comparison with more traditional, scientifically based public health skills such as critical appraisal and epidemiological knowledge. Persuasion, negotiation and influence were looked at in more detail, and the notion of principled negotiation was proposed as an approach to improve the potential outcomes of negotiation. Six influence strategies were discussed and their potential use in public health considered. On balance, preventative and preparatory strategies seemed to offer the greatest likelihood of being both effective and acceptable.

The nature of power in organisations and the use of power in improving public health were considered. Power was seen as a complex and important phenomenon for the public health workforce to understand. Different models of power were described, and each had in common a consideration of how power was enacted and the resources that could be used.

Finally, some common problems in communication, such as a dissonance between the intended message and the received one, were explored using simple models of communication.

GOING FURTHER

Etzioni, A (1975) *A Comparative Analysis of Complex Organizations* (rev. edn). New York: The Free Press.

This is a classic analysis of sources of organisational power. Looking at power from an organisational perspective, Etzioni makes a distinction between coercive power, remunerative power and normative power.

Fisher, R, Ury, W and Patton, B (1999) *Getting to Yes: Negotiating an Agreement without Giving in* (2nd edn). London: Random House Business Books.
This is a classic book in the field of negotiation that is accessible and full of practical guidance and advice. It explains what successful negotiation is all about.

Handy, C (1993) *Understanding Organizations* (4th edn). Harmondsworth: Penguin.
Handy's book is an essential reader if you are interested in organisational theory and behaviour. The book is organised into three parts: the first part consists of seven chapters that focus on a range of organisational concepts such as organisational theory, motivation leadership style and contingency theories. Chapter 4 is particularly relevant, as is Chapter 10. The second part focuses on concepts in action, and the final part provides a summary of the book as a whole.

Corcoran, N (ed.) (2007) *Communicating Health, Strategies for Health Promotion*. London: Sage.
Drawing on recent research and health promotion theory, this book provides some interesting reading in relation to communication. Chapter 1 in particular considers a wider range of theory related to communication.

chapter 6
Leading Communities Collaboratively
Susie Sykes

Meeting the Public Health Competences

This chapter will help you to evidence the following competence for public health (Public Health Skills and Career Framework):

- Level 5(1) Collaborate with others effectively to improve population health and wellbeing;
- Level 6(1) Engage and work collaboratively with a range of people and agencies to improve population health and wellbeing;
- Level 6(2) Identify opportunities and develop structures to take forward approaches to improve population health and wellbeing, including making use of partnership working;
- Level 6(6) Review the effectiveness of collaborative working and make recommendations for improvement;
- Level 6(a) Knowledge of the models and principles of leadership and their application;
- Level 6(b) Knowledge of the principles and methods of partnership working and the benefits which collaboration can bring to the health and wellbeing of the population;
- Level 7(2) Engage and influence others in and beyond own organisation to improve population health and wellbeing;
- Level 7(3) Lead others across projects or programmes to improve population health and wellbeing;
- Level 7(7) Review the effectiveness of collaborative working and make the necessary improvements;
- Level 7(a) Understanding of the principles and methods of partnership working and the benefits which collaboration can bring;
- Level 8(1) Lead on improving population health and wellbeing within and/or across organisations;
- Level 8(6) Review collaborative working and put in place the necessary improvements;
- Level 8(7) Build and sustain capacity and capability through individual, team, organisational and partnership development;
- Level 8(a) Understanding of the models and principles of leadership and their potential use in improving and protecting health and wellbeing and in motivating colleagues and partners.

This chapter will also assist you in demonstrating the following National Occupational Standards for public health:

- Lead others in improving health and wellbeing (PHP45).

In addition, this chapter should be useful in demonstrating Standard 11(c) of the Public Health Practitioner Standards:

Standard 11. Work collaboratively with people from teams and agencies other than one's own to improve health and wellbeing outcomes – demonstrating:

c. awareness of:

    i. principles of effective partnership working.

Overview

This chapter will help you consider what the term 'leadership' means when working in a community context. It will explore what is meant by the term 'community' and the different models for working in and with communities to improve health and wellbeing, including an examination of the principles of participation and empowerment. In particular, it will help you consider what is meant by the term 'community leadership' and the opportunities and challenges that such an approach offers.

Public health practitioners are regularly required to work in partnership with individuals, projects and agencies in community settings in order to improve the health and wellbeing of that community. This chapter will help to identify the potential challenges that may exist in this kind of work, and enable you to identify strategies for overcoming these challenges.

The activities in this chapter will focus on:

- developing clarity about the nature of the term 'community';
- understanding different approaches to community work;
- exploring the concept of empowerment as applied to whole communities;
- developing an understanding of the challenges of community leadership.

This chapter uses theory, tools and case studies to explore leadership in a community context. After reading this chapter you will be able to:

- appreciate the drivers behind the political positioning of community and the changing definitions of the term 'community';
- identify a range of models and definitions of community, community work and community development;
- articulate the distinction between community-based and community development work, and the notions of participation and empowerment;
- identify the potential challenges that exist in developing community leadership.

Why communities?

In seeking to understand the relevance for public health of communities and community-led or community-based work, it is useful to begin by briefly examining the place that communities have had in the recent political agenda. The concept of communities has always had a place within public policy, although the way that the term has been conceptualised, the connotations attached to it, the expectations of communities and the role they can and should play in society – and in particular, in developing and delivering public policy – has shifted according to political perspectives and dominant ideologies. Principles of socialism, for example, emphasise equality, shared ownership and responsibility for others, while the neoliberal principles of the New Right under Margaret Thatcher placed the individual as the primary and central policy focus, encouraging competition and acceptance of inequalities. With this came an increasingly dominant view of some communities being deserving and others undeserving.

The 'Third Way' ideology of New Labour sought to bring together neoliberal principles of the free market with principles of social justice and equality, thus placing community at the interface between the state and individuals (Ledwith, 2005), and seeing communities as both the problem and the solution. Thus, New Labour developed a whole stream of policies with a community focus, seeking to tackle social and health inequalities and build community cohesion: 1997 onwards saw a first wave of initiatives with a community focus such as Health Action Zones, New Deal for Communities and Sure Start, along with a new rhetoric of empowerment, involvement and participation. Ensuing policies such as *The NHS Plan* (Department of Health, 2000), *Choosing Health: Making Healthier Choices Easier* (Department of Health, 2004a), *Creating a Patient-Led NHS: Delivering the NHS Improvement Plan* (Department of Health, 2005) *Our Health, Our Care, Our Say* (Department of Health, 2006b) and the Local Government and Public Involvement in Health Act 2007 included a central commitment to the idea that communities were best placed to know and understand their own needs, and that they should have a say in how services and public health should be delivered.

The central place of communities in government policy looks set to continue under the Conservative–Liberal Democrat coalition government's commitment to the concept of the 'Big Society', with its emphasis on transferring power from central to local government and giving communities more powers to run local services. However, the ideological impetus is different. The 'Big Society' is intended to replace rather than complement the 'big government' (Cabinet Office, 2010), with action at a local level being seen as an alternative to action taken by state institutions and public services.

ACTIVITY 6.1

Consider a public policy that has influenced your work in recent years.

Where were communities located within this policy?

Were they seen as the recipients of a service or initiative, or the route through which a service or initiative could be delivered?

How far was the policy informed by local voices?

Comment

The shifting focus on communities in health policy is, in part, a result of the increasing acknowledgement of the social, economic and environmental context of health (Wanless, 2004), the recognition that health inequalities are the result of social inequalities, and that the reduction of health inequalities requires, among other things, creating and developing healthy and sustainable places and communities (Marmot, 2010). Marmot demonstrates the extent to which the health and wellbeing of individuals is influenced by the places in which they live, not only because of the physical environment, but also because of the social networks and social capital that communities can offer. He also demonstrates the link between the extent of people's participation in their communities and psychosocial wellbeing.

Defining 'community'

In order to understand the place of community in both policy and practice, it is necessary to unravel the term and explore the different definitions and ways in which it is used. It remains an ambiguous and sometimes contested term which has different meanings according to the context and motivations of the user. Indeed, in the 1970s Plant (1978) identified more than 90 different definitions being used in the literature of the time.

For some, rather than produce an all-encompassing definition of the concept, it has been more useful to identify different types of communities. One frequently presented set of categories is that of geography, culture and social stratification (Naidoo and Wills, 2009). In this categorisation, geography refers to those communities that are based on neighbourhood or locality; communities of culture are those groups of people that share common cultural traditions and bonds; and communities based on social stratification are groups that come together because of a common interest which is the result of the way in which society is structured, such as the 'working class' community.

For others, identifying the attributes that cut across different types of community is more important. Clark (1996) outlines a true community as one that offers the individual the '3 Ss': significance, security and solidarity. However, this does focus on the positive attributes of the concept without acknowledging the diversity, inequality and occasional conflict that can exist within communities. Taylor (2003) usefully identifies three ways in which the term is used: as a descriptive term to describe those who share common interest; as a normative term to denote a set of values and conditions that underpin how we should live; and as an instrumental term which combines elements of the previous two, while attaching agency and collective action to the term.

ACTIVITY 6.2

Think about a community with which you work.

What are the characteristics of this collection of people that makes you call them a community?

Do they refer to themselves as a community?

What positive things do you think that being a member of this community brings to people's lives?

Can membership of a community ever impact on people's lives in a negative way?

Comment

Often, populations that we are tasked to work with as public health practitioners have been labelled as 'communities' by policymakers or professionals, and this may not represent how the population actually feels about itself. Communities that are defined as such by outsiders may feel resentful about the term, resulting in less co-operation and support and hiding the differences and existence of marginalised groups within it. Communities that have defined themselves as communities are more likely to be made up of networks and organisations that are bound together in some way. As such, they are likely to be more organised, resolve conflict internally and be more articulate in making demands on service providers (Emmal and Conn, 2004).

The term 'community' often suggests a place of cohesion and safety, of shared values, norms and aspirations. It may be viewed from a systems perspective, with the community composed of individual members and sectors which have different characteristics and functions within society, operating within specific boundaries to meet goals for the good of the whole (Homan, 2008). However, it is also important to acknowledge the complexity of divisions and conflict that can exist within communities. Ledwith (2005) warns us that forces of exploitation and discrimination permeate communities. Where communities are based on shared values and ideals, those who do not share those values and ideals and choose to live their life in a different way may face isolation or exclusion from the community they grew up in or identify as being theirs. Communities, then, can become places of oppression with entrenched traditions and hierarchies that trap people into particular roles, and where the majority voice is heard but the voice of minority groups is not given a platform and becomes drowned out. Professionals and commentators often talk about the needs of a community without recognising that the individuals within it may have different and sometimes conflicting needs.

Working with communities

Not only is there confusion and contention around the term 'community', but there is considerable confusion around the definitions and usage of many of the concepts associated with work in and with communities. This may be due in part to the adoption within policy of terms and ways of working that once belonged to the more radical work of community development and community action (Ledwith, 2007). With this application in more mainstream settings, the meanings and understandings of the terms have changed. Table 6.1 provides a set of characteristics for a number of different terms related to community work.

Table 6.1 Community activity in multidisciplinary public health: concepts and definitions

Community action	Collective action by local communities, with increasing control by people over the area in which they live. This may involve campaigning in response to a specific issue of concern.
Community development in health	A process whereby people, both individually and in groups, exercise their right to play an active role in developing health services.
Community involvement	Entails both consultation and participation with local people in developing policies and local services to improve their health. It shares many features of community participation, but usually takes place over a longer period of time and is more involved.
Community participation	The process of ensuring that community members have a say in decision-making about issues that affect them. This may be done through formal partnerships, public meetings, forums and consultation documents, focus groups, surveys, community councils, advisory committees or appointing representatives to health committees.
Capacity-building	Developmental work that increases the abilities of a community or organisation to take action or provide services. This may include skills and confidence-building, building infrastructures, improving organisation and procedures, etc.
Civic engagement	Active participation in the institutions of civil society, including signing petitions, contacting local officials and attending public meetings.
Consultation	A slightly higher level of involvement than giving of information. People may be asked for their views of an issue of policy and may be offered choices in what should be done. There is no opportunity for people to develop their own ideas or have any real power to make decisions.
Empowerment	A social process that promotes the participation of individuals, organisations and communities in actions with the goal of increased individual and community control, political efficacy, improved quality of life and social justice.
Social capital	The features of social life, such as networks, norms and social trust that facilitate co-ordination and co-operation for mutual benefit. It represents the degree of social cohesion that exists in communities.

Source: Adapted from Handsley (2007)

The approaches to community focused work are numerous, and the blurring of the boundaries between them makes it difficult to categorise them clearly. Thomas identified five different strands or approaches to community work in the 1980s:

1. community action or the collective action of communities to challenge sociopolitical and economic structures and decisions;

2. community development, emphasising self-help and mutual support;

3. social planning concerned with the assessment of community needs and problems, resulting in systematic planning of strategies to meet them;

4. community organisation involving the joint working of different community or welfare agencies to promote joint initiatives; and

5. service extension, which involves extending services into the community to make them more accessible (Thomas, 1983).

While this framework was based on a review undertaken in the 1980s, the distinctions remain relevant today.

ACTIVITY 6.3

Consider the different community-focused work being undertaken in the area in which you live or work.

Can you identify them according to the strands provided by Thomas?

Can you identify any other approaches to community work that is not covered by Thomas' framework?

Other categories of community work are offered in the literature, with Twelvetrees (1991) making the distinction between 'professional' and 'radical' community work. 'Professional' community work emphasises attempts to promote self-help and improve the effectiveness and appropriateness of service delivery; and 'radical' community work emphasises the potential to shift the framework of existing social relations and challenge oppressions at their source. A frequently made point of distinction that is important for health professionals and public health practitioners to appreciate is between 'working in communities' and 'working with communities' (Labonte, 1998; Green and Tones, 2010). In work *in* communities, the community represents the setting or target for work and is associated with 'top-down' initiatives, where aims and processes are determined outside the community. Work *with* communities includes involving the community in identifying and addressing its own needs, and is associated with participatory 'bottom-up' approaches. Initiatives that fall within this category draw on the principles and values of community development as a model.

Definitions of community development, like other terms in this field, are diverse and sometimes contradictory. The National Occupational Standards for Community Development Work define it as:

> *a long term value based process which aims to address imbalances in power and bring about change founded on social justice, equality and inclusion.*

(2009, p4)

– with a process that includes working with people to:

- *Identify their own needs and aspirations.*

- *Take action to exert influence on the decisions which affect their lives.*

- *Improve the quality of their own lives, the communities in which they live, the societies of which they are a part.*

(2009, p4)

Therefore, as a model it is both value-based and political, seeking to tackle power imbalances and question the status quo in order to challenge oppression and empower both individuals and communities. Community development has a long history with its roots in colonialism, when colonial administrators attempted to develop basic education and social welfare in British colonies through self-help. Following the work of the community development projects in the 1970s, the notion became associated with more radical approaches (Smith, 2006). One of the key influencing forces of community development approaches is the work of Brazilian educationalist Paolo Freire (1973). His emancipatory principles and techniques were based on the understanding that change would be generated by oppressed people through the development of critical consciousness-raising, or an awareness of their own oppressed situation leading to collective action.

The recent dominant position of community development within mainstream policy reflects a rather different and less radical position, and a case could be presented to argue that many state-sponsored community development initiatives are in fact better described as community-based, rather than truly reflecting the traditional community development model. As Shaw argues:

> *[C]ommunity development has been, and continues to be, subject to competing rationalities, inhabiting a position at the intersection of a range of opposing ideas, traditions, visions and interest – claimed by the right, left and centre with equal enthusiasm.*

(Shaw, 2008, p33)

Table 6.2 distinguishes between community-based and community-development models, and Table 6.3 provides a summary of activities associated with community development.

Leading for Health and Wellbeing

Table 6.2 Characteristics of community-based versus community-development models

Community-based	Community-development
Problem, targets and action defined by sponsoring body	Problem, targets and action defined by community
Community seen as medium, venue or setting for intervention	Community itself the target of intervention in respect to capacity building and empowerment
Notion of 'community' relatively unproblematic	Community recognised as complex, changing, subject to power imbalances and conflict
Target largely individuals within either geographic area or specific subgroup in geographic area defined by sponsoring body	Target may be community structures or services and policies that impact on the health of the community
Activities largely health-oriented	Activities may be quite broad-based, targeting wider factors with an impact on health, but with indirect health outcomes (empowerment, social capital)

Source: Adapted from Labonte (1998). Reproduced with kind permission.

Table 6.3 Community development worker activities

Typical activities in which a community development worker might be involved

Building trust and relationships	Accessing resources
Networking	Capacity-building
Providing leadership and co-ordination	Facilitating and promoting self-help
Developing new community-based programmes	Raising public awareness
Community profiling	Mediating conflict
Motivating individuals and encouraging participation	Liaising with statutory organisations
Managing volunteers	Managing finances
Challenging oppression and discrimination	Liaising with the media
Contributing to strategy development	Evaluating, monitoring, report writing
Needs assessment	

A model of work with communities which has gained currency in recent years has become known as the 'asset approach' or 'Asset Based Community Development' (Kretzmann and McKnight, 1997). This argues for a move away from the more traditional 'deficit' approach, which focuses on the problems, needs and deficiencies in a community that result in services and interventions being designed to fill the gaps. Rather, it focuses on what the community does have in place, valuing the capacity, skills, knowledge, connections in a community and how these can be built upon in order to ensure that a community meets its potential (Improvement and Development Agency (IDeA), 2010). The approach builds on the concept of salutogenesis (Antonovsky, 1979), which highlights the factors that create and support human health and wellbeing rather than those that cause disease. The asset approach does not replace investment in services or tackling the structural determinants of health,

108

but aims to build a better balance between service delivery and community-building, as illustrated in Table 6.4.

Table 6.4 Moving from a deficit approach to an asset approach

Where we are now – the deficit approach	Where an asset way of thinking takes us
Start with deficiencies and needs in the community	Start with the assets in the community
Respond to problems	Identify opportunities and strengths
Provide services to users	Invest in people as citizens
Emphasise the role of agencies	Emphasis the role of civil society
Focus on individuals	Focus on communities/neighbourhoods and the common good
See people as clients an consumers receiving services	See people as citizens and co-producers with something to offer
Treat people as passive and done to	Help people to take control of their lives
'Fix people'	Support people to develop their potential
Implement programmes as the answer	See people as the answer

Source: IDeA (2010, p12). Reproduced with kind permission.

Empowerment

Despite the ambiguities that surround the concept of community development and other forms of work with communities, there are two concepts that can be seen to be dominant: empowerment and participation. As with many of the other terms used in this field, many definitions are applied to both of these according to context and the views of the writer. Empowerment has been defined both as a process and as an outcome, but one often-quoted definition is provided by Gibson as:

> *a social process of recognizing, promoting and enhancing people's abilities to meet their own needs, solve their own problems and mobilize the necessary resources in order to feel in control of their own lives.*

> (Gibson, 1991, p359)

As a definition that focuses on the process of empowerment we are able to identify a number of key stages, which begin with a recognition of one's own situation and an acknowledgement of any inequity, social injustice or oppression. This builds on the work of Freire's (1973) and his concept of critical consciousness-raising (as outlined above). Following this comes a stage of bringing people from similar situations together or mobilising the community, so that the community itself is in a position to identify and prioritise its own needs and go on to identify appropriate responses to those needs.

However, this is not a straightforward linear process, but a complex set of reflections and actions that results in a fundamental shift of power towards those previously excluded, marginalised or oppressed. Dalrymple and Burke (2006) offer a useful framework, suggesting that empowerment should be viewed as operating on three levels: feeling, ideas and action. The level of feeling relates to the feelings of an individual in relation to their own powerlessness. At this level the individual begins to makes links between personal and social issues, while building feelings of self-worth and confidence. At the level of ideas a change occurs, whereby there is a decrease in self-blame and a raised awareness that structural factors play a part in our situation; that once this is identified, there is an increased belief in the possibility and need to change things. At the level of action we see a move away from the personal to the political: this is about the individual acting, in either a micro or macro way, to ensure that they influence any decisions that are made that affect them.

ACTIVITY 6.4

Identify an intervention that claims to empower people.

To what extent did it act on the levels of feeling, ideas and action?

To what extent did it result in a transition of power?

While Dalrymple and Burke's framework refers to the individual, it is important to acknowledge that the concept of empowerment can be equally applied to whole communities, although key to this remains making the link between the personal (whether on an individual or community basis) and the structural.

Lavarack (2004) offers an analysis of community empowerment and represents it as a five-point continuum model (Figure 6.1).

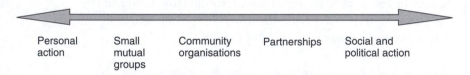

| Personal action | Small mutual groups | Community organisations | Partnerships | Social and political action |

Figure 6.1 A continuum of an empowered community

Source: Lavarack (2004, p48). Reproduced with kind permission.

Lavarack presents each stage in this continuum as an outcome in its own right, as well as progression along the continuum. While each community may be at a different starting point along this line, the process often begins with the individual and the development of their own power and ability to act. Once there is a critical mass of individuals operating at a level of personal action, it is possible to bring like-minded and motivated people together into small mutual groups to begin the process of social cohesion and collective action. Community organisations represent a progression whereby groups become more structured with a leadership function, and begin to move beyond looking at the needs of individuals within a group and begin looking more broadly at the needs of a community as a whole. The next stage is the coming together of similarly conceived organisations to work effectively in partnerships with other organisations in order to pursue shared goals, putting competing interests to one side. According to this model, a community is truly empowered when individuals, collectives and partnerships are able to influence decision and policymaking through social and political action. This is a hard level to reach, but Lavarack argues that the skilled practitioner or community development worker can play an important role in moving a community along this continuum.

Empowerment is another, once radical term, which has been appropriated by the mainstream in recent decades. With this comes the danger that it will lose its agenda for social change and become a euphemism for social control: rather than seeking to challenge the status quo, the process is about subtle victim-blaming and getting people to do what we want of them. Empowerment as a concept presents the practitioner with some very real dilemmas and challenges.

ACTIVITY 6.5

Consider the following points.

Is empowerment another way to get people to do what we want?

Does everyone want to be empowered?

What negative consequences could come with empowerment?

How do you measure empowerment?

Comment

The process of empowerment begins with a reflection by an individual on their place in their wider community and society in order to identify social injustice, powerlessness and oppression. This, it is argued, is necessary in order for an individual to move beyond their current position and ensure a more just and 'empowered' place in society. This self-reflection and acknowledgement of previously unrecognised powerlessness or oppression may represent a very difficult process for people and may have negative consequences, such as the destabilising of relationships.

Participation

Using the model of the empowered community presented above, it is clear that participation of individuals and communities is a key component of the empowerment process; however, a distinction in the terms needs to be made clear. While community members may influence how an intervention is designed or delivered through participation in the process, this does not automatically mean that they can be described as an empowered community that is able to work for and effect political and social change.

Strategies for the involvement and participation of patients and the public have underpinned much health policy in recent years, and participation has been seen to have particular relevance to tackling health inequalities. There is clearly a rationale for such strategies, including that ensuring services and interventions are designed and delivered in response to local need, and increased accountability and transparency, reflecting the democratic process as well as the personal outcomes for those involved. Understanding the different levels of participation is key to understanding the complexity and different usage of this concept. Several authors have presented typologies of the term which present different levels of participation. Often this has been done in a hierarchical way according to the amount of power-sharing and the degree of influence over decision-making, thus making a distinction between consultation, participation and empowerment (Wills, 2009). Popay (2010) provides a model that links increased participation to service, social and health outcomes (Figure 6.2)

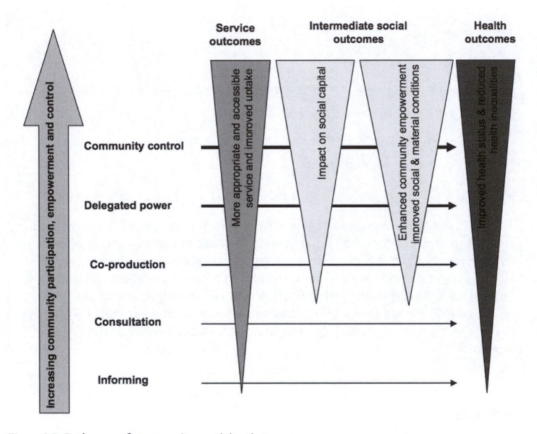

Figure 6.2 Pathways of community participation

Source: Popay (2010). Reproduced with kind permission from Springer Science+Business Media.

This model distinguishes between the following:

- informing people or the giving of information about decisions already made;
- consulting people or asking people to select a preference from a predetermined set of options;

- co-production, whereby clients or service users work alongside professionals as partners to create and deliver services;

- delegated power, which gives the public a limited amount of decision-making power for a particular policy or service but with the proviso that this power is not permanent and can be withdrawn; and

- community control, whereby a community-based organisation is given total responsibility and therefore accountability for a particular service or area of activity.

The framework provides a theoretical link proposing that community engagement approaches which operate at the level of informing only have a marginal impact on the health of those involved, but may play a role in making services more accessible. Those approaches that offer co-production, delegated power or total community control are seen to lead to more positive health outcomes, as well as social outcomes such as increased levels of social capital. While this and other models of participation present different types of participation as a hierarchy, achieving the highest level of participation should not necessarily be seen as the ultimate goal. Rather, the context and objectives need to be carefully assessed in order to decide when it is appropriate or sufficient to operate at the level of informing, and when there is sufficient times-cale, commitment, resources and need to work towards a higher level of participation and even community control.

Leading communities

In reviewing the nature, approaches and underpinning principles of public health work with and in communities, it is important to consider the role and place of leadership. The public health competencies that frame the work of public health practitioners call for leading others across projects or programmes to improve population health and wellbeing, and for engagement with and influencing others in and beyond one's own organisation to improve population health and wellbeing. McNaught (2009) argues that although the practice of community leadership within a postmodern context departs at many critical points from more traditional and radical approaches to community development, community leadership is an essential resource for galvanising communities around health issues, and is therefore an important public health skill.

As outlined in Chapters 1 and 2, traditionally, leadership is seen to be about change and the ability to overcome resistance to a particular course of action (Leach and Wilson, 2000). In his editorial on leadership for health promotion and public health, Catford (1997) identifies the two distinguishing features of a leader: first, a responsibility for significantly changing the attitudes, behaviours and actions of a large number of people; and second, an ability to achieve this to a degree beyond that expected of somebody purely in a management or hierarchical position. As mentioned previously, one of the key challenges of leadership in communities is that it requires leadership across a network of organisations, as opposed to leadership within one organisation or structure (McNaught, 2009). This network is likely to consist of organisations that embody different organisational cultures and different priorities and visions. However, beyond these very real challenges lies a more fundamental question of how this 'top-down' concept of change according to a leader's vision fits with the kinds of work *with* communities outlined above, which embrace 'bottom-up' approaches with a commitment to the principles of participation and empowerment.

In seeking to provide answers to this question, much can be learnt from the experience of the local government context. With the transition of public health from the primary care trust to the local authority setting, perhaps it is even more fitting that we look in this direction for learning. Community leadership was a constant theme in New Labour's programme of local government reform, beginning soon after coming into power with the White Paper *Modern Local Government: In Touch with the People* (Department of the Environment, Transport and the Regions, 1998), which presented the commitment to community leadership. The theme went on to be developed in policy and guidance documents throughout the New Labour administration. The vision of this concept represented a move away from a more classical definition of leadership and involved local government focusing on the needs of communities over its own interests, working in partnership rather than exercising complete control, working towards change and responding to local aspirations (Lowndes, 2004).

The concept of community leadership as embodied within the local government agenda is complex, but was usefully represented by the Audit Commission (2003), as summarised in Figure 6.3.

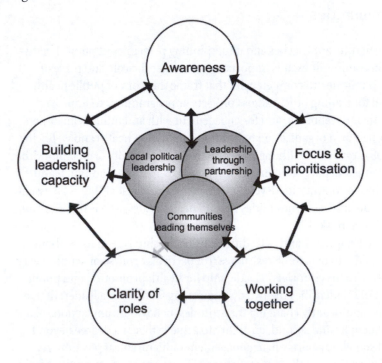

Figure 6.3 The Audit Commission model of community leadership

Source: Adapted from the Audit Commission (2003) and Madden (2010a) Reproduced with kind permission.

According to this model, community leadership is made up of three overlapping fields:

1. local democratic leadership – or the bringing together of people in order to develop a vision for their area;

2. leadership through partnership – such as the Local Strategic Partnerships and other collaborative bodies; and

3. communities leading themselves – which refers to the building of capacity and social capital within communities.

This building of capacity and social capital is required in order for communities to participate effectively in the first two fields (Madden, 2010b). In this model the local authority is not required to exercise leadership 'over' communities; instead, it acts as an agent of its community, with the authority to lead not assumed from the electoral process but from being legitimised by communities through a process of expressing their own needs and wants, and brokering agreement in the inevitable case of conflict (Sullivan *et al.*, 2006). Thus the role contains an apparently contradictory position: the local authority has to hand over a degree of power to the community and make a commitment to community involvement and empowerment, while retaining accountability for ensuring that the overall good of the community is advanced – even when this may contradict the expressed needs or wants of the elements of the community that are engaged. These positions were reflected in early evaluations, which showed that there were two distinct interpretations of the term 'community leadership' as it was being applied through local government – the role of the local authority as a strategic leader and as a democratic champion (Sullivan, 2008).

It could be argued that to see real transfer of power requires more than a generation, and that despite the end of the New Labour administration it is too early to see the outcome of its community leadership vision. However, evaluations have shown that the strategic leadership element of community leadership has been implemented more successfully than the inter-agency collaboration and community engagement elements. Community engagement in particular as been identified as the element of community leadership which has been least successfully applied, and remains the biggest challenge (Sullivan *et al.*, 2006).

Towards a more sophisticated understanding of community leadership

Thus, we can see more sophisticated understandings of the concept of community leadership coming to the fore. Madden (2010b) describes this as *'transformational leadership'* – at once both leader and follower in a process that involves shared change, and transforms both the leader and the follower. Alternative conceptualisations of the term include 'catalytic leadership' (Luke, 1997), whereby leaders think strategically but also have the skills to engage others in productive collaboration, and 'distributed leadership' (Hartley and Lawton, 1998; Gronn, 2002), where one charismatic figure is not required to possess all the leadership skills, rather, where a number of senior officials have overlapping and complementary skills to represent the complex governance context.

Doyle and Smith (2009) go on to explore leadership as something that arises out of social relationships and comes from how people act together to make sense of a situation rather than depending on one person. This notion of shared leadership means that in one situation, an individual may be influential because of their position or the skills that they possess, while in another situation, it may be somebody different. Thus there is a shift in expectation from one person having a vision and the skills to realise it, to looking internally at a group's capacity to create that vision and act upon it, with movement from focusing on position to process, individual activity to social interaction, and order to conversation. Doyle and Smith (2009) are clear that this comes with challenges. First, the focus on process can cause the product or outcome to be neglected. Second, the focus on groupwork may cause the exceptional skills of individuals within it to be overlooked. Third, the complex commitments of shared leadership make it a model that some find difficult to embrace. Finally, models of leadership are culturally specific, and so what may be viewed as appropriate in one group may not be in another. However, despite these challenges, this movement beyond the classical characteristics of leadership enables us to view leadership in away that is not as far removed from the some of the principles of community development as might be assumed at first. Table 6.5 compares the characteristics of classical and shared leadership.

Table 6.5 Classical and shared leadership compared

Classical leadership	*Shared leadership*
Displayed by a person's position in a group or hierarchy	Identified by the quality of people's interactions rather than on their position
Leadership evaluated by whether the leader solves problems	Leadership evaluated by how people are working together
Leaders provide solutions and answers	All work to enhance the process and to make it more fulfilling
Distinct differences between leaders and followers: character, skill, etc.	People are interdependent. All are active participants in the process of leadership
Communication is often formal	Communication is crucial with a stress on conversation
Can often rely on secrecy, deception and pay-offs	Values democratic processes, honesty and shared ethics. Seeks a common good

Source: Doyle and Smith (2009), drawing from material in Nemerowicz and Rosi (1997, p16). Reproduced with kind permission.

Challenges of community engagement

The experience of attempting to embed community leadership within the local authority has much to teach the public health practitioner. In particular, the challenges of pursuing the public engagement field of this agenda are important, and reflect some of the difficulties that were faced by NHS staff in implementing the Patient and Public Involvement agenda. Foremost among these challenges is the difficulty of ensuring that the community is fairly represented, and that those groups most likely to be disengaged and excluded from society and its political systems are provided with an appropriate route through which to have their voice heard. A further challenge is to ensure that the community is not solely represented by people who are already comfortable and familiar with negotiating their way around local democratic systems. Ensuring that the mechanisms through which the public is engaged are relevant and appropriate is key: attempts to run community engagement events as scaled-down, formal meetings using the language and format of professionals will not effectively engage the members of the community that are most excluded. Effective community engagement requires creative thinking and a requirement to work on terms and in ways that are likely to be less comfortable to the professional.

A further challenge is getting the community to want to be engaged. In their research, Sullivan *et al.* (2006) identified a combination of reasons expressed as to why people were not motivated to participate in local democracy:

- an ignorance of local authority structures and responsibilities;

- a culture of contentment whereby people felt things were 'good enough';

- a feeling that engagement events were for a 'certain kind of person' or would be dominated by a single issue; and

- a feeling that the agenda and decisions had been made already by the local authority.

While there are no easy answers as to how these challenges can be overcome, there must be a recognition and acceptance that working with communities requires an investment of time and a commitment to building relationships, trust and routes for effective communication. If the intention is to lead communities collaboratively, then there also must be a reflection on the distribution of power and how it can be more evenly shared.

Chapter summary

In this chapter we began by considering the changing face of community within the political agenda and some of the drivers behind its political positioning. From this, the definitions of the term 'community' were examined in order to aid our understanding of the place of communities in both policy and practice. The range of definitions illustrate the complexity of the term, and help us to see that while for some the term denotes cohesion and safety, it also may encompass divisions and conflict.

Moving on to look at working with communities, several of the many different approaches were identified. In particular, the distinction between community-based and community development work was explored. Key to community development are empowerment and participation, both of which were defined and examined within a practice context.

Finally, against this backdrop, the concept of community leadership was introduced, which was presented as an essential resource for galvanising communities around health issues, while acknowledging the departure from and potential contradiction to more traditional and radical community development (McNaught, 2009). Lessons from work within a local authority context were reflected upon, suggesting the need for a move away from traditional models of 'leadership over' to transformational leadership or the role of democratic champions. This is not without its challenges, and these were explored.

GOING FURTHER

Craig, G, Mayo, M, Popple, K, Mayo, M and Taylor, M (2011) *The Community Development Reader*. Bristol: Policy Press.
This book contains a series of articles from key authors in the field of community development, mapping out the changing context of community development and illustrating the principles that underpin it, as well as the challenges that it faces.

Laverack, G (2009) *Public Health: Power, Empowerment and Professional Practice*. Basingstoke: Palgrave Macmillan.
This book introduces ideas of power and empowerment within public health practice, with practical ideas for transforming power relations with individuals and communities. The case studies are particularly useful.

Green, J and Tones, K (2010) *Health Promotion: Planning and Strategies* (2nd edn). London: Sage.
Chapter 9 provides a useful introduction and overview of different approaches to working with communities.

Butcher, H, Banks, S, Henderson, P with Robertson, J (2007) *Critical Community Practice*. Bristol: Policy Press.
This book presents a particular model for community practice from a critical perspective. Chapter 6 offers some thought-provoking ideas around organisation leadership and management when working within this framework.

chapter 7

Leading at a Local Level
John Harvey and Rhonda Ware

Meeting the Public Health Competences

This chapter will help you to evidence the following competences for public health (Public Health Skills and Career Framework):

- Level 5(5) Promote the value of population health and wellbeing and the reduction of inequalities in various teams or agencies;
- Level 6(5) Promote the value of health and wellbeing and the reduction of inequalities across settings and agencies;
- Level 6(d) Knowledge of theories and approaches of managing people and their application;
- Level 7(1) Manage programmes or projects to improve population health and wellbeing;
- Level 7(3) Lead others across projects or programmes to improve population health and wellbeing;
- Level 7(8) Build and sustain capacity and capability through individual and team development;
- Level 7(9) Have insight into own behaviour within teams and in various settings;
- Level 7(h) Knowledge of the design and implementation of performance management;
- Level 8(1) Lead on improving population health and wellbeing within and/or across organisations;
- Level 8(h) Understanding of the design and implementation of performance management.

This chapter will also assist you in demonstrating the following National Occupational Standards for public health:

- Provide leadership for your team (M&L_B5);
- Provide leadership in your area of responsibility (M&L_B6);
- Lead others in improving health and wellbeing (PHP45);
- Develop and sustain cross-sectoral collaborative working for health and wellbeing (PHS09);
- Provide leadership for your organisation (M&L_B7).

In addition, this chapter will be useful in demonstrating Standards 11 and 12 of the Public Health Practitioner Standards:

Standard 11. Work collaboratively with people from teams and agencies other than one's own to improve health and wellbeing outcomes – demonstrating:

a. awareness of personal impact on others;
b. constructive relationships with a range of people who contribute to population health and wellbeing;
c. awareness of:

    i. principles of effective partnership working;
    ii. the ways in which organisations, teams and individuals work together to improve health and wellbeing outcomes;
    iii. the different forms that teams might take.

Standard 12. Communicate effectively with a range of different people using different methods.

Overview

This chapter looks at a health improvement leadership framework as a template for understanding the skills needed to lead public health in a local environment. The arguments are structured around three dimensions: professional, political and people. Key topics include credibility, public health as core business and performance management within the department.

This chapter will help you understand the challenges of leadership locally and to have a set of practical tools both to lead in the political environment and manage a department.

The activities in this chapter will focus on:

* appreciating the strengths and weaknesses of different approaches to leadership and their potential use in improving population health and wellbeing;
* improving your management skills and personal credibility;
* exploring the opportunities for public health from political change (such as the Localism Bill in England) and the ethical dilemmas faced;
* experiences of performance appraisal and identifying examples of good practice;
* experiences of succession planning and identifying the need for succession planning at a local level.

After reading this chapter you will be able to:

* identify key elements of public health leadership and the need to balance duties across three dimensions – political, professional and people;
* develop an understanding of what public health leadership at a local level entails and identify key challenges;
* understand the performance management cycle and consider the implications for managing and improving performance at a local level;
* consider the importance of succession planning and implications at a local level.

What have we learned about leadership and management?

The distinction (or not) between leadership and management was discussed in Chapter 1. Hunter quotes Mintzberg rejecting this distinction, stating that *managers have to lead and leaders have to manage* (Hunter, 2007, p4). This is an important debate as there has been, rightly, considerable criticism of both management and leadership in the UK NHS. A report published in October 2011 by the Care Quality Commission (2011) highlighted the deficiencies in care for older people in NHS hospitals. Asked to comment, the spokesperson for the Royal College of Nursing said the problem was partly *lack of clinical leadership*. By this, she meant a reinvention of the ward sister role, but her comments echo a common cry in respect of transforming the England NHS: namely, for stronger leadership.

In local public health teams the same issue comes to the fore: what is wanted is leadership. Hannaway *et al.* define leadership as *the art of getting things done by enabling others to do more than they could or would do otherwise* (in Hunter, 2007, p153). As discussed in Chapter 2, Hannaway and colleagues set out a framework for the Leadership for Health Improvement Programme, identifying three key domains (Hannaway *et al.*, 2007). The improvement of health improvement systems (A in Figure 7.1) is the first and sets the context. Improvement knowledge and skills (B) is the second, and focuses on the study and practice of enhancing performance, and leadership (C) is the third area.

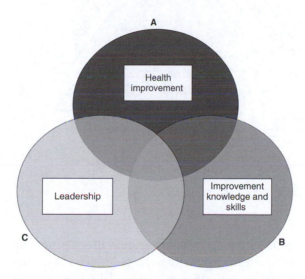

Figure 7.1 Leadership for Health Improvement Programme Framework

Source: Adapted from Hannaway *et al.* (2007)

Local leadership: balancing duties

A duty is an obligation and can come from different sources. It could be a moral obligation, for example. In this context it is a result of one's particular place in life, that is, a member of a profession, the job itself (leading and managing) and the organisation. In the UK, the director of public health is the leader for public health in the local environment.

The vision of the role of the director of public health in England, as set out in the UK government White Paper *Healthy Lives, Healthy People* (Department of Health, 2010b), envisages that the director of public health will be the principal adviser on all health matters to the local authority. The director of public health in this strategy will be responsible for health improvement, addressing local inequalities in health outcomes, and addressing the wider determinants of health. They will work in partnerships. Directors of public health are expected to discharge a professional duty to keep their skills up-to-date and to ensure that their staff are similarly well trained. In this national vision the skills of the director of public health will ensure that there is a competent, local, multidisciplinary public health workforce with strong professional leadership at its heart.

In practice, these responsibilities and duties fall into three broad dimensions, as illustrated in Figure 7.2.

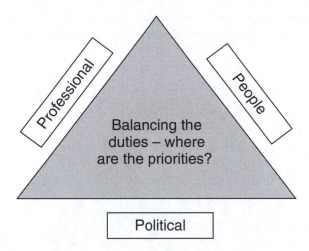

Figure 7.2 Three dimensions of local leadership

The first dimension, *political*, entails the duties set out within the organisation and the wider political environment. Organisations are political bodies. The structure defines boundaries and levels, with differentiated specialisation, power and rewards. Interestingly, these political and structural divisions encourage informational divisions, which distort the content and flow of information (Hodgkinson and Sparrow, 2002). The move of local public health departments or teams into the local authority places the team squarely in a local political culture, where democratically elected members decide priorities and control the budgets.

The second dimension is the *professional*. The Faculty of Public Health Standards Committee published a guide in 2002 called *Good Public Health Practice*, which states that public health professionals must:

- *practise good standards of public health, as described in this guidance, and with particular reference to the nine key areas of activity and their necessary competencies;*

- *make sure that individuals and communities are not put at risk; and*

- *work within the limits of their professional competence.*
        (Faculty of Public Health Standards Committee, 2002, p10)

This guidance reflects the General Medical Council (GMC) guidance for doctors (GMC, 2006) which includes duties to:

- protect and promote the health of patients and the public;

- provide a good standard of practice and care;

- keep their professional knowledge and skills up-to-date;

- recognise and work within the limits of their competence; and

- work with colleagues in the ways that best serve patients' interests.

The third dimension, *people*, is based on a duty of care and respect. This includes the public as the ultimate customer, partners and staff.

Each of these three dimensions can be mapped onto the Leadership for Health Improvement framework, as illustrated in Table 7.1.

Table 7.1 Attributes of leadership on three dimensions

Dimension	Domain in Leadership for Health Improvement framework
Professional:	
Develops health programmes and services and reduce inequalities	A
Encourages and implements evidence-based practice	A
Seeks to create new evidence and to translate evidence into practice	B
Sets up measurement to demonstrate impact and gain insight into variation	B
Develops quality and risk management within an evaluation culture	B
Political:	
Earns and retains the confidence of politicians and others	A
Operationalises a strategic vision of the future	A
Prioritises and focuses on key issues and leverage points in the health improvement system	A
Builds relationships and works collaboratively across organisational boundaries	C

Challenges thinking and encourages flexibility, creativity and innovation	C
Sees whole system and any counterintuitive linkages between them	B
People:	
Communicates clear vision direction and roles	C
Continuously increases capacity to deliver the health improvement agenda -	A
Nurtures a culture in which leadership can be developed and enabled in others	C
Demonstrates mastery of management skills	C
Spreads improvement ideas and knowledge quickly and widely	B

The professional dimension

Beginning with this dimension – perhaps the key to local leadership – there is an unspoken recognition that a leader must be credible. To be the local public health leader the individual must be seen to be knowledgeable (if not wise), have an excellent track record of achievement and be able to persuade others of the strength of the public health case: or importantly, the population health view on other aspects of corporate business.

What's the evidence?

Rychetnik *et al.* considered the credibility of evidence of public health interventions. They noted that public health interventions are *complex, programmatic and context dependent* (2002, p119). Similarly, they argued that evidence must be able to encompass and reflect such complexity in order to sufficiently discriminate between the success or failure of the process of evaluating intervention, and the success or failure of the intervention itself. Furthermore, the evidence should be able to help discern whether the intervention was inherently defective, or simply poorly delivered.

They concluded:

> *The appraisal of evidence about public health interventions should encompass not only the credibility of evidence, but also its completeness and its transferability. The evaluation of an intervention's effectiveness should be matched to the stage of development of that intervention. The evaluation should also be designed to detect all the important effects of the intervention, and to encapsulate the interests of all the important stakeholders.*
>
> (Rychetnik *et al.*, 2002, p125)

Being knowledgeable

Knowledge is critical, and falls into four main categories:

1. knowing the place and people;
2. knowing the strengths and weaknesses of public health theory and practice;
3. knowing what is happening outside your area (and the UK); and
4. knowing the business.

KNOWING THE PLACE AND PEOPLE

Local public health leadership starts with investigating and understanding the place for which you have responsibility, and the people who live there. This is not simply reading the latest health profile from the Association of Public Health Observatories, useful though this is. It requires getting out and about to see and listen, reading the relevant local strategies and reports (such as economic analysis and sustainable community strategies) and visiting key institutions such as schools or services.

KNOWING THE STRENGTHS AND WEAKNESSES OF PUBLIC HEALTH THEORY AND PRACTICE

Contrary to the perception that we like to give as specialists in a scientific field, the truth is that we do not have all the answers. So we need to choose the arguments we take on, especially around the predicted impact of public health programmes. A lot of public health activity is driven by central agendas and based on little evidence of effectiveness. The old paradigm of knowledge>attitude>behaviour change has been replaced by a more subtle understanding of social marketing and behaviour change technologies. Life-course, resilience and place have taken on huge importance, as understanding of the determinants of health moves steadily forward from an unhealthy reliance on the medical models of public health. (Life-course theories are discussed in Chapter 1 of *Measuring Health and Wellbeing* in this series.)

KNOWING WHAT IS HAPPENING OUTSIDE YOUR AREA (AND THE UK)

Public health networks are potentially large, even global, but in practice often confined to a region at best. In the NHS in England, directors of public health would meet in local regional groups, where often they were treated as competitive siblings – not the most conducive approach to enhancing leadership. Indeed, the folly of treating neighbouring areas as 'benchmarks' (i.e. how does my patch compare to the others in the cluster or region?) creates false comfort or discomfort. It is far more productive to seek out and be familiar with good practice in other regions and countries. A good example is the environmental justice movement:

The concept of 'environmental justice', as it is currently understood, is largely the product of the activities of a network of community groups in the USA. These groups have resisted the siting of polluting factories and waste sites in predominantly black neighbourhoods and indigenous people's reservations. This movement – which has taken a civil rights and social justice approach to 'environmental' problems – has been aided by a substantial US academic literature which has documented the extent and causes of environmental injustices.

(Economic and Social Research Council Global Environmental Change Programme, 2001, p5)

KNOWING THE BUSINESS

This is about contributing to and understanding the values and corporate goals of the organisation of which the public health team is a part, and of the partners. Historically, health promotion units and currently, health improvement teams, have preferred to go about their business without necessarily understanding what others saw as the core business. (This issue is discussed below) The essence of the argument here is that if one is in a leadership role in an organisation whose main business is to spend several hundred million pounds on commissioning healthcare, then it is imperative to have a critical knowledge of healthcare commissioning. If the organisation has the spread of functions, such as a unitary local authority, then the public health leader needs to get to grips with the purpose and challenges of those functions. There is a bonus here, as it enables the public health team to identify the opportunities for synergy.

Having a track record of achievement

Interviewers at appointment panels are encouraged to ask questions about specific achievements: for example, 'Tell me about the most challenging project you completed'. It ought to be unlikely that someone is appointed to a position of leadership without a substantial track record. The track record brings two strengths to the potential leader. Whether it is in the management of change or in delivering a particular success in public health practice, confidence comes from experience. Confidence also comes from having the breadth and depth of knowledge discussed above. The other strength is readiness to innovate.

Innovation is about doing something different in the local working environment, not necessarily inventing a totally new approach. An example of a substantially different approach, although not new and which requires strong leadership, is programme budgeting and marginal analysis (discussed in Chapter 1 of *Measuring Health and Wellbeing* in this series). The adoption of this health economic technique has been promoted through the road test report published by the York and Humber Public Health Observatory (Kemp *et al.*, 2008). The conclusions from this pilot work were that programme budgeting and marginal analysis has the potential to change patterns of service, but it needs to be linked into the commissioning or service redesign process. The participants valued different perspectives and viewpoints and this was a significant benefit, giving considerable enthusiasm to make programme budgeting and marginal analysis part of the commissioning.

This approach to public health reaches out to communities, facilitates their involvement and enhances their capacity to respond to priority health issues.

What's the evidence?

Dickinson *et al.* (2011) discuss the role and value of leadership in addressing problems in relation to priority-setting in healthcare. They look at the technical and rational aspects of priority setting, the challenges of relational leadership and the presentation of priority-setting as a 'wicked issue'. They distinguish technical and adaptive responses depending on whether the barrier is tame, such as lack of evidence, or wicked, such as unrealistic stakeholder expectations. They conclude that there are issues relating to the degree of autonomy that a local leader has, and around the support that they need in taking this agenda forward. This analysis points to the potential and limitations of key leadership concepts such as 'sense-making' and 'framing'.

Being able to persuade others

One of the understated attributes listed in the person specification for a director of public health is 'good presentational skills (written and oral)'. However, the main essential communication skills are described as *excellent oral and written communication skills (including dealing with the media) and effective interpersonal, motivational and influencing skills* (Faculty of Public Health, 2007). The leader must be able to convince the partners that it is worth investing in programmes or projects aimed at improving health and wellbeing. For example, life-course theories are accepted as a major contribution to understanding how adult health and wellbeing is influenced by what happens in the early years of life. The Marmot Review has emphasised the pre-eminent place of Early Years programmes in tackling inequalities (World Health Organization (WHO), 2008). Given the role and responsibilities of local authorities in education and children's services, the challenge here is to persuade NHS commissioners to invest adequately in these services and, perhaps more importantly, to adopt a valid instrument to measure outcomes.

Another example is the role of place in influencing health and wellbeing. Again, local authorities in the UK are increasingly orientated to this conceptually. Indeed, this is a distinct topic in the Leadership Centre for Local Government programme. You should be familiar with reports such as a WHO Europe publication entitled *Environmental Burden of Disease Associated with Inadequate Housing* (Braubach *et al.*, 2011).

ACTIVITY 7.1

Looking back at Table 7.1 and the five attributes under the professional dimension, ask yourself the following.

Could I prepare three slides for the health and wellbeing board on what I know to be really important, and one slide listing issues that I need to research, remembering to demonstrate:

- knowing the place and people;
- knowing the strengths and weaknesses of public health theory and practice;
- knowing what is happening outside my area (and the UK);
- knowing the business?

Comment

Despite the comment about 'the easy approach' above, a good map, for example of child poverty indicators by small area, will illustrate the essence of the social determinants and identify the most vulnerable areas. Life-course theory is not commonly understood, yet can be simply illustrated. An example of effective practice in another place linked to your slide on public health theory will be relevant. If the theme is children, then effective support at family level for vulnerable families might be a good example.

Knowing the business is about showing the links or synergy with the responsibilities and functions of the partners. If the theme is children, then links to Children's Centres, primary schools, youth offending teams, etc. will be powerful – especially if you can focus on changes in outcomes.

The political dimension

Organisations are political bodies (as discussed in Chapter 3). Handy (1999[1976]) points out the obvious: that organisations are made up of people and act as communities. A number of negative words are conjured up: 'cliques', 'cabals', 'personality clash', 'conflict' and 'competition'. As he says:

> *[T]he challenge for the manager is to harness the energy and thrust of the differences so that the organisation [which may be the public health department] does not disintegrate but develops.*

(Handy, 1999 [1976], p291)

At a local level a public health leader needs both to understand the politics of the organisation and the partner organisations, and to work out strategies to harness the differences within and without. The movement of public health to local authorities (in England) and to a democratic political process are increasingly significant. In this context, the shifting of public health to a position where it is seen as core business and managing in a way that is consistent with, and influential within, the corporate (and partnership) ethos, is important. Understanding and navigating the 'political game' could be seen as a key political leadership challenge.

What's the evidence?

Mintzberg (1983b) describes 13 political games commonly found in organisations. These can be briefly described as follows.

Insurgency game

Revolution from the bottom, which aims to sabotage the intentions of superiors. Often has a transactional child–parent basis.

Counter-insurgency game

Played by the senior managers or executives as they fight back against the insurgents. Has a parent–child basis, so there are more rules and boundary setting and sanctions.

Sponsorship game

Building power through attaching oneself to a powerful superior. This might require reciprocal favours.

Alliance-building game

Building power through peer networks, or attaching oneself to a colleague who is perceived to be powerful.

Empire-building game

Building a power base through coalitions of subordinates. Internal competition, then, is between groups or teams rather than individuals.

Budgeting game

Building power by taking control of resources. This is what gives finance directors and their staff such enormous and disproportional influence in the NHS.

Expertise game

This is played by people with expertise, where they use their knowledge and skills more for their own gain than for that of the organisation. The expertise may be feigned: it relates to the power of having or dispensing information.

Lording game

Played with the power of one's position, flaunting one's authority, getting staff to do one's bidding.

Line versus staff game

A game between line managers who are managing the day-to-day working of the organisation, and the staff who seek to spread best practice or develop standard operational procedures, for example. It may be a game aimed at defeating a potential rival.

Rival camps game

This often happens between departments, such as commissioning and finance, where there are different goals and interests, and it is easy to blame the other team.

Strategic candidates game

This may happen when there are different options under consideration and groups of people support one or other idea. Often, one side will try to discredit the other through misinformation.

Whistle-blowing game

Where an insider leaks information (perhaps to the press). This may be done due to principles, naivety or with specific political intent, such as to discredit a rival.

'Young Turks' game

It may involve one or several people and aggression is the major characteristic. It appears in leadership challenges and attempts to change strategic direction.

Public health leaders need to be cognisant of these in order to navigate the political territory successfully.

Leading within organisations

As mentioned previously in this book, in England, local public health departments which were part of Primary Care Trusts (PCTs) are moving into local authorities. Although this is seen as a major change, directors of public health have been joint appointments for several years and are expected to show leadership in both cultures and within strategic partnerships. However, the relocation into local government offices and day-to-day accountability to the chief executive (an accountability which is presumed) is a very different situation. There are different ways of doing the business, and different attitudes to targets and performance management, but the main challenge is the relationship with members: the democratically elected councillors. This relationship, like any other, requires time and mutual respect to develop. They differ from non-executive directors in the NHS trusts in three important respects. They have an overt political affiliation, represent a local constituency of real people with varied agendas, and are the decision-makers.

ACTIVITY 7.2

What opportunities does the Localism Bill in England present to public health?

Think about your own context and the opportunities that this may create (or has created).

What might be the potential disadvantages?

How might you maximise the opportunities presented and minimise any disadvantages?

A summary of the Localism Bill (and its passage through Parliament) can be accessed at: **www.communities.gov.uk/publications/localgovernment/localism-plainenglishguide** (Department for Communities and Local Government, 2008).

Taking the four main provisions (new freedoms and flexibilities for local government, new rights and powers for communities and individuals, reform to make the planning system more democratic and more effective, and reform to ensure that decisions about housing are taken locally), what public health goals could be better reached by taking advantage of the different measures?

Conversely, what threats are there to public health goals?

How would you, as the local public health leader, manage the opportunities and threats?

Comment

The context of public health leadership is change – a reality in any public sector organisation. In 2011 the English government introduced a Bill on Localism, which sets out to provide the four main provisions listed above.

These measures can be seen as an opportunity for public health. The local leader will want to understand what can be done further to address the social determinants in the light of the proposals. These proposals will have different impacts across local government. The opportunity is to plan for and build in health to the built environment. It would be worth researching what can be done from a public health perspective. The threats are the possible adverse impacts due to undue influence of short-term economic factors on local politics, with loss of green spaces and poorly designed housing development.

Whatever the organisational and inherent political context, the public health leader will aim to achieve two main leadership goals:

• to place the public health department at the core of the corporate business;
• to manage the department in a way that is consistent with, and influential within, the corporate ethos.

Public health as core business

If the definition of public health is accepted as *the science and art of preventing disease, prolonging life and promoting health through the organised efforts and informed choices of society, organisations, public and private, communities and individuals* (Winslow, 1920), then it could be argued that any organisation is, or should be, a public health organisation. However, the argument here is that public health staff can contribute to a multidisciplinary approach to all functions of the organisation, and that their skills can be seen to be indispensable.

In order to illustrate this argument, consider this situation. The main business of NHS commissioners (most recently, PCTs) is to spend a large amount of money to commission and pay for healthcare for the defined population. The legacy of service configuration in most areas of England is an inefficient use of too many hospital sites. For several years strategic plans have been made – and successfully achieved in a few places – to rationalise service provision and recognise the need to concentrate some specialist services, in order to sustain the quality of the outcomes. A good example of the rationale is stroke care. Recent reviews of quality of care in the NHS emphasised the failure to achieve international standards in the care of people with stroke: this led to proposals to create tertiary-level centres to provide first-line care. What role should the director of public health play? They will want to be part of the planning, assuring commissioners that the evidence is robust and supports the proposals. Then they should take on a public and professional advocacy role to promote the plans and focus attention on the quality issues. The benefit is credibility as a corporate player, and consequentially credibility when advocating public health initiatives.

Managing in a way that is consistent with, and influential within, the corporate ethos

When thinking about the corporate role and visible performance of the department, it is useful to have groups of interrelated headings. These can serve also as a framework for thinking about managing people and programes. The starting point is values, and the rest should derive from those values. This can be represented as a 'values cube', where each face of the cube represents a specific aspect relating to values (as illustrated in Figure 7.3). The first face is values, and the other five faces of the cube are clarifying and articulating functions, optimising the structure, setting objectives in line with the business plan, communication and performance review.

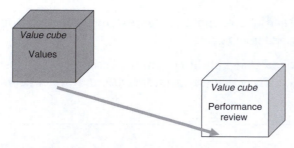

Figure 7.3 A values cube

Building on the different elements of the values cube, a number of key activities emerge.

Set the values and mission to reflect the corporate vision

In discussing leadership and values, Pendleton and King conclude that:

> [L]eadership reexamines the procedures that organisations follow and ensures that these procedures fully reflect the organisation's vision and values – that they prepare it for its future challenges, rather than merely reflect its former glories.
>
> (2002, p1354)

Public health leaders should work to ensure that the core values for improving health are embedded into the organisation vision.

Mant (1984) describes two sorts of people, and indicates that one sort (ternary thinkers or builders) make better leaders. They are not focused on 'shall we win', but on the 'what's it for?' question – that is, the task or purpose (Mant, 1984, quoted in Handy, 1999[1976]: p108). These leaders will have a clear set of values that are related to the purpose. Ideally, the values of the organisation will be such that the public health team can define its aims within that framework. By and large, when given space to define vision and values, public sector organisations come up with similar concepts.

Clarifying and articulating functions

This is an important basic step. It is achieved by a paper for an audience of other directors and their departments, which might use the three aspects of public health described by the faculty as a basis, but will set out the main functions such as need assessment, health intelligence and community development within that framework.

Agreeing objectives in line with the corporate business plan

It follows that a director must have a business plan for the department which matches the corporate strategy and operational plans. This should be agreed with the senior management team, so there is clear understanding of the department's priorities and how they contribute to the corporate priorities. The plan should contain a risk assessment, with a statement of proposed mitigating actions.

Optimising the organisational structure

The organisational structure of the department is very important to the members of the department, but should reflect the overall structure of the organisation. One key thing to avoid is having two people in different departments holding the same or overlapping remits. There are always efficiencies to be had by avoiding duplication and encouraging matrix working.

Communication

The director is the source of messages for the public health team about the corporate goals, performance and any planned change. They must show leadership in communicating these to the team and by listening attentively, knowing what messages to take up to the senior management team.

Performance management

The public sector has undergone a journey deep into performance management since the late 1990s. This has led to the emergence of an inappropriate use of indicators in some areas, which may not truly reflect the impact of public health programmes. The challenge for the public health leader is to propose better measures and have them accepted. Each department objective should have a meaningful outcome measure to enable the impact to be evaluated.

What's the evidence?

Handy (1999[1976], pp107–15) suggests that a leader must take into account four different influences when confronting any given situation. These are *the leader*, *the subordinates* and *the task*, which all depend to a greater or lesser extent on *the environment*. Handy proposes a 'best fit' approach, which maintains that the leader will be most effective when the requirements of the first three (leader, subordinates and task) align or 'fit'. The scale he proposes to measure the fit is linear and runs from 'tight' to 'flexible'.

In the context of this section, the influence of the environment is critical. Handy lists six key aspects of the environment: these include the power position of the leader in the organisation and the organisational norms. The complicating factors include the variety of the tasks. The leader's fit on the scale will depend on factors such as their values and need for certainty.

This approach helps us to understand the complexity of the leadership role, and provides an analytical approach to enable the leader to achieve a 'best fit' wherever possible.

Within partnerships

Standards for Better Health, originally published in 2004 (Department of Health, 2004b, p17), included a specific standard, C22, on the level of partnership working (in England), which required:

> *healthcare organisations (to) promote, protect and demonstrably improve the health of the community served, and narrow health inequalities, by:*
>
> - *cooperating with each other and with local authorities and other organisations;*
>
> - *making an appropriate and effective contribution to local partnership arrangements, including local strategic partnerships, and crime and disorder reduction partnerships.*
>
> (Department of Health, 2004, p17)

The Healthcare Commission subsequently set out criteria requiring healthcare organisations to cooperate with, engage and support local partnerships – for example, the local strategic partnership (LSP) and have a representative on such partnerships; and requiring PCTs to agree a set of local priorities to improve health and narrow health inequalities, developed in collaboration with the council and other healthcare organisations. Also, there were requirements to develop priorities for health improvement and narrowing health inequalities, reflecting the findings and recommendations of a local health needs assessment, including equity and health impact audits and national public service agreement targets. This provided a useful set of parameters for the focus of local public health leadership in the partnership context, namely:

- engaging and supporting the partners;

- leading prioritisation;

- enhancing and interpreting the joint strategic needs assessment;

- ensuring that relevant equity and impact audits are done frequently;

- and advocating outcome targets that are locally useful.

The criteria set by the then Healthcare Commission included:

- healthcare organisations ensuring they cooperate with, engage and support, local partnerships, for example the local strategic partnership, and have a representative on such partnerships;

- PCTs agreeing a set of local priorities to improve health and narrow health inequalities, developed in collaboration with the council and other healthcare organisations;

- priorities for health improvement and narrowing health inequalities, reflecting the findings and recommendations of a local health needs assessment, including equity and health impact audits and national public service agreement targets (IDeA, 2009).

This sets a useful set of parameters for the focus of local public health leadership in the partnership context, namely:

- engaging and supporting the partners;

- leading prioritisation;

- enhancing and interpreting the joint strategic needs assessment;

- ensuring that relevant equity and impact audits are done frequently; and

- advocating outcome targets that are locally useful.

Returning to focus on the values cube presented earlier in this chapter, the six faces of the cube (setting values, clarifying and articulating functions, optimising the structure, setting objectives in line with the business plan, communication and performance review) are equally pertinent to partnerships, as illustrated in the Children's Trusts case study.

Case Study: Children's Trusts

Section 10 of the Children Act 2004 required local authorities in England to make arrangements to promote co-operation between themselves, named 'relevant partners' and others as appropriate, to improve the wellbeing of children in the authority's area.

The implications of this duty were that partners needed to work together to build Children's Trusts. These would be shared arrangements centred around the needs of the child, which provide strategic direction through a Children's Trust board. The purpose of a Children's Trust in meeting the requirements of the Act
would be set out in a local children and young people's plan. The plan was required to satisfy criteria set out in guidance and had to include:

- a statement of improvements planned for children and young people;
- vision and principles;
- assessment of need;
- priorities and key actions;
- resources to be applied to those priorities (arrangements for commissioning);
- a statement of how workforce reform supports outcomes;
- arrangements for reporting (performance management monitoring and review);
- arrangements for governance and Trust development (duty to co-operate);
- links with other statutory plans.

In one London borough the director, as the local leader for public health and executive lead for the wellbeing of children and young people, was able to influence the arrangements and goals in three key ways.

First, by defining the primary function, and therefore membership of the Trust board, as commissioning. This was an important principle: it meant that providers were not included on the board, which would set the strategy and overall priorities articulated in the children and young people's plan, monitor outcomes and hold to account contributors to the wellbeing of children and young people.

Second, through needs assessment and an annual public health report devoted to children and young people, the director could argue for the following priorities:

- introduce long-term care management for children and young people with complex needs;
- develop new roles to support children and young people with mental health issues;
- identify children with rising Body Mass Index (BMI) early;
- support parents in the Early Years.

Third, the director was able to contribute to the communication strategy, both through an emphasis on talking to children and young people, and taking a lead role in a series of workshops or seminars for staff working for all the partners.

Stewart (2002, p8) argues that leadership in and across partnerships is needed to inspire vision enthusiasm and commitment. For Stewart there are three categorisations of leadership:

1. leadership as designed and focused;

2. leadership as implied and fragmented; and

3. leadership as emergent and formative.

A designed and focused leadership such as the mayoral model may be more decisive, but only if there is representational legitimacy. A fragmented collaborative approach to leadership may offer an attractive compromise on leadership, but it is subservient to external policy influence and dominated by bureaucratic arrangements. Formative leadership is pragmatic and depends on implementation for legitimacy, but the fragility of partnership structures and processes may mitigate against achieving the desired goals.

The tasks associated with leadership in partnership change according to the maturity of partnership. Stewart concludes that *leadership in co-ordinating partnerships is evident in support for the practice of working together – assembling funding packages, establishing joint teams, aligning objectives* (2002, p8).

ACTIVITY 7.3

The local strategic partnership members are asked by the local authority to write letters of support for an application to build a casino complex on a brownfield site. The argument is that the casino will provide jobs and bring a huge boost to the local economy. As a public health leader (director of public health), you receive a letter in your own right, and the chair of the PCT, as a member of the local strategic partnership board, has also received one. In consultation with the chief executive, the chair of the PCT writes and sends a strong letter of support.

What research will you do to decide how to reply?

What are the important topics?

Look at the evidence before answering the next questions.

Who might you speak to as part of that exercise?

Will you discuss the issues with the chief executive and chair?

If your research leads you to believe that the casino is not good for the public health and wellbeing, how will you proceed?

Comment

This exercise throws up two dilemmas.

1. Is the director truly independent? Will they take a line that is opposed to those to whom they are managerially accountable?
2. What is the balance between the economic argument, which may bring benefits in terms of employment and income, and the public mental health argument, which identifies the adverse impact?

You will want to think through the strategy for submitting any opinion that is opposed to the proposed development. Using personal networks will be vital. Organisations such as the Royal College of Psychiatry will have a view on the impact of gambling on individuals and families.

The people dimension

Successful staff management is key to success as a leader within the organisation, department and wider health economy as a whole. Planning for the future and ensuring arrangements to develop capacity as well as capability and succession planning are critical activities. How will you know that the leadership and management activity is successful? How will you measure success? These are important questions that need to be answered. An understanding of organisational culture, change management and performance management and succession management are important attributes within the people dimension. Organisational culture and change management are explored in Chapters 3 and 9; here, we will focus on performance management and succession management.

Performance management

According to Armstrong, performance management is *a process which contributes to the effective management of individuals and teams in order to achieve high levels of organisational performance* (2009, p618). It establishes both a shared understanding about what is to be achieved, and an approach to leading and developing people that will ensure it is achieved.

Performance management has a number of elements, and should encompass performance improvement and staff development (Sisson and Storey, 2000). Through a process of setting objectives, review and follow-up, the management (and work) of individuals and groups is linked to the corporate objectives. At its best, performance management is a tool to ensure that managers manage effectively. Through performance management, managers ensure that their people or teams:

- know and understand what is expected of them;
- have the skills and ability to deliver on those expectations;
- are supported by the organisation in developing the capacity to meet those expectations;
- are given feedback on their performance; and
- have the opportunity to discuss and contribute to individual and team aims and objectives.

At its worst, it is a tick box exercise and fitted into the 'day job'.

Performance management is also about ensuring that managers themselves are aware of the impact of their own behaviour on the people that they manage, and are encouraged to identify and exhibit positive behaviours.

MANAGING PERFORMANCE WITHIN A DEPARTMENT

First, we will look at some of the issues to do with structure and setting objectives, then we will discuss the vital concept of self-awareness before looking at the performance management and improvement of individuals.

Structure. There are some essentials to leading a department. First, ensure the following:

- that you have a structure that meets the needs of the business;

- that it is able to deliver the outcomes required; and

- that there is a clear structure for the public health department, with clear functions, reporting lines and accountability.

The objectives of the organisation and the department need to be understood to ensure that personnel with the relevant knowledge and skills are recruited and retained. Regular review of the organisation chart will help to identify whether the department is still 'fit for purpose'.

Setting objectives consistent with the business plan. The importance of this cannot be over-emphasised. All individuals working in the department need to know the organisation's business vision, goals and objectives, and be signed up to achieving them. Objectives clarify the expectations of individuals and therefore are a useful management tool, enabling performance to be measured. Within the department, objectives may be set for teams and individuals: set high expectations that are a challenge, but not too challenging; conversely, do not set them too low so that people are not motivated and become bored. Articulate these expectations and ensure that they are understood. Anderson (2010) identifies that individuals will be more motivated when they can relate their activities and objectives to their business. He goes on to clarify further the role of the leader within performance management as that of a conductor of a corporate orchestra, directing and balancing overall cohesion with individual flair (Anderson, 2010, p139).

Knowing your team. The most motivated members of a team are those that feel valued, that their roles are taken seriously and that they have a sense of belonging. Valuing staff should be demonstrated by getting to know each individual: what makes them tick, their values and beliefs, and personal or health circumstances that may get in the way of fulfilling their role. It is important to recognise these and then support staff to remove or reduce these barriers.

Supporting your team when needed. Be aware of your management or leadership style. Do you empower your staff, or do you like to maintain control? In a highly political environment, a dictatorial or control style is often highly exercised and an empowering model is less likely to be used. In essence, leaders should use a range of management styles to lead their teams. The styles used may depend on the individual with whom you are communicating.

Managing performance. In order to assess the department's performance, clear objectives according to the business plan need to be agreed and set out. Objectives need to be SMART:

Specific
Measurable
Articulated (agreed)
Realistic; and
Timely.

Objectives should be set for the public health organisation as a whole, then for specific departments, since the requirements from each department may be quite specific, and then for individuals. Performance assessment is usually done on a yearly basis through performance development review or appraisal, and usually includes a mid-year (or quarterly) review. There are supposed to be no surprises during this process: that is, if there are performance issues, these should have been realised and discussed already.

ACTIVITY 7.4

Think about your own experience of being appraised and of having appraised others.

Can you identify any potential problems that you faced or needed to be overcome?

Can you identify those elements that seem to constitute good practice?

What are the implications of this for performance appraisal?

Comment

It is likely that you will have identified time as a key problem: time to prepare the performance review paperwork, to identify objectives in the first place and to carry out the performance review itself. This is a common problem, and sufficient protected time is vital if the process is not going to end up as a tick-box paper exercise. Having clearly agreed targets and standards against which to assess performance outcomes, together with constructive feedback and opportunities to review and agree personal development plans, contributes to effective practice. In many organisations the human resources department provides support in the form of 'appraisee and appraiser' training, and acts in an advisory capacity as a resource to managers and staff at all levels.

Recent developments in performance management have seen the introduction of new tools such as 360-degree feedback, which can be used in a number of ways. These tools gather feedback on an individual from a number of sources, typically including colleagues, direct reports and peers. Supporters claim that this gives managers and individuals better information about skills and performance as well as working relationships, compared to more traditional appraisal arrangements based on line managers' assessment (Chartered Institute of Personnel and Development (CIPD), 2011). Such tools also can be very useful in identifying areas for performance improvement. In addition, coaching and mentoring can be used to enhance and improve individual performance.

Succession management

It is important to recognise that for an organisation to succeed, leadership encompasses planning for the future. Succession management refers to identifying and developing potential successors in an organisation. The key in succession management is to create a match between the organisation's or department future needs, and the aspirations of individual employees.

Leadership in the local context is challenging, but can be very rewarding. The key issues have been discussed with an emphasis on knowledge: knowing the business, knowing the team and especially knowing yourself. Leadership is as much about learning as any other aspect of a professional role.

Chapter summary

In this chapter we began by revisiting the need for leadership, before considering a framework for leadership for health improvement that focuses on health improvement, leadership and improvement knowledge and skills. Local leadership and the need to balance duties across three dimensions – political, professional and people – led to some deliberation on how these might relate to the leadership for health improvement framework. Exploring these dimensions further highlighted a number of key aspects of public health leadership.

From the professional dimension, these included being knowledgeable (in a number of ways), having a track record of achievement and being able to persuade others. Focusing on the political dimension, understanding the politics of the organisation and partner organisations, the democratic political process, positioning public health so that it is seen as core business, and managing in a way that is consistent with, and influential within, the corporate (and partnership) ethos, were viewed as important within organisations and across partnerships. The people dimension has a focus on the successful management of staff and the delivery of corporate and health improvement objectives. Performance management, the appraisal and performance review process, and the use of tools such as 360-degree feedback to identify areas, were discussed. In addition, succession planning and management were viewed as critical to the long-term success of public health.

This chapter concludes by arguing that leadership at a local level is challenging: knowing the business, the team and yourself are key.

GOING FURTHER

Handy, C (1999[1976]) *Understanding Organisations*. Harmondsworth: Penguin.
    Chapter 4 on leadership, and Chapter 10 on politics and change, give helpful insights into the types of leadership and the political context of organisations.

Hunter, DJ (ed.) (2007) *Managing for Health.* Abingdon: Routledge.
    This book tackles many facets of leadership and gives the reader a window into a wealth of practical knowledge relevant to leading public health.

chapter 8

Leading and Managing Projects
Vicki Taylor and Vivien Martin

Meeting the Public Health Competences

This chapter will help you to evidence the following competences for public health (Public Health Skills and Career Framework):

- Level 5(3) Plan, implement and review specific aspects of health improvement projects;
- Level 6(3) Co-ordinate programmes or projects to improve population health and wellbeing;
- Level 6(c) Understanding of theories and models of project management and their application;
- Level 7(1) Manage programmes or projects to improve population health and wellbeing;
- Level 7(3) Lead others across projects or programmes to improve population health and wellbeing.

This chapter will also assist you in demonstrating the following National Occupational Standards for public health:

- Manage a project (M&L_F1);
- Manage programme of complimentary projects (M&L_F2).

In addition, this chapter will be useful in demonstrating Standard 10d of the Public Health Practitioner Standards:

Standard 10. Support the implementation of policies and strategies to improve health and wellbeing outcomes – demonstrating:

d. the ability to prioritise and manage projects and/or services in own area of work.

Overview

This chapter will help you to develop your thinking about managing projects and, in particular, managing projects to improve health. We will consider the key dimensions of time, budget and the quality of outcomes and why it is important to keep these in balance. We will also consider what is needed to manage a project and how you can plan and manage the key stages of a project, including implementation, and how you can monitor and control progress towards achieving the project objectives. We will consider how you might use the 7 Questions framework to identify and manage a relatively straightforward project, and introduce some of the tools to manage more complex projects. Finally, we will consider some key features of successful projects and look at some common problems experienced in projects.

The activities in this chapter will focus on:

- developing clarity about the nature of public health projects;
- understanding the different stages of a project;
- exploring the tools that can be used in each stage of a project;
- developing a critical awareness of the importance of people in projects and, in particular, stakeholders.

Public health practitioners are regularly required to manage projects. They are involved in setting up, planning, implementing and handing over a wide range of different types of projects. In this chapter the main features of a project and the key stages will be explored in order to help you to identify ways to manage projects more effectively. A number of useful tools that can be used at each stage are introduced.

After reading this chapter you will be able to:

- identify the main features of a public health project;
- understand the different stages in a public health project;
- understand and use some of the main project management tools and techniques;
- understand and manage better the relationships with the internal and external stakeholders of the public health project(s) in which you are involved.

What is a project?

Often, the word 'project' is used to describe a wide range of activities, some of which are very large and complex, whereas others are small and straightforward. Projects can be distinguished from routine activities or wider aspects of change because they have specific objectives, limited timescales and a budget based on an estimate of the costs. Usually, they also have an identified project manager who reports to someone responsible for the budget: this project manager is often either 'part-time' and carrying out this role alongside their normal routine work, or for larger projects, might be seconded to the project for its duration. Most public health practitioners are involved in projects, and many might be managing several projects at the same time. Managing projects is an integral part of public health work and these projects are usually expected to lead to improvements in public health.

What are public health projects?

Public health projects can be wide-ranging and broad in scope, but most will address the determinants of health and be concerned on some level with improving health. Some will focus on addressing the wider social and economic determinants of health. Others might address specific aspects of the physical environment in which people live and work, their health behaviours, social factors or the range of health services (Longest, 2004), or a complex combination of these.

ACTIVITY 8.1

Think of a public health project that you know well, or in which you have been involved.

What is it that makes it a project?

Are projects different from other work? If so, in what ways do they differ?

Spend a few minutes thinking about these questions and jot down your answers.

How does a programme differ from a project?

Comment

The word 'project' can be used to describe many types of public health work. Maylor (2005, p4–6) suggests that while there are many different definitions of project, there are some commonalities. For example, there is consensus on the following:

- projects involve a process, with constraints such as time, resources and deliverables that define and limit the process;
- projects are comprised of focused activity, often involving change;
- projects are goal-oriented.

Public health projects often have a considerable number of stakeholders, all of whom require information about progress and opportunities to contribute to shaping the direction of the project. You might have thought about projects that are commissioned and involve one or more partners, or projects that are jointly funded. Public health projects typically involve a wide range of different stakeholders with different expectations and interests in the project. You also may have identified that public health projects are frequently managed and co-ordinated through a steering group or partnership board, with representatives from key stakeholders.

In addition, you might have thought about projects that are commissioned and involve one or more partners, or projects that are jointly funded. Public health projects often have a considerable number of stakeholders, all of whom require information about progress as well as opportunities to contribute to shaping the direction of the project. Public health projects also typically involve a wide range of different stakeholders with different expectations of, and interests in, the project. Moreover, you may have identified that public health projects are frequently managed and co-ordinated through a steering group or partnership board, with representatives from key stakeholders.

All projects are time-limited, and this is what distinguishes them from other areas of work. All projects have specific beginning and endpoints (Frame, 2003), although these may not always run as planned. One of the key points in managing projects, rather than programmes, is their nature: *It is usually a one-off non-repeated activity that is intended to achieve specified objectives and quality requirements within a time limit* (Martin, 2002, p248).

A programme may have a limited timescale too, but will usually last for several years – much longer than most projects, unless the project is a major building development. Usually, a programme will settle into routine activities for its duration, rather than move through the typical key stages of a project. These key stages are often referred to as the 'project life cycle', and will be discussed later in this chapter.

Dimensions of a project

The British Standard for Project Management (BS60794 1996) defines project management as:

> *The planning, monitoring and control of all aspects of a project and the motivation of all those involved in it to achieve the project objectives on time and to the specified cost, quality and performance.*

The UK Association of Project Management provides a definition for project management as:

> *The planning, organisation, monitoring and control of all aspects of a project and the motivation of all involved to achieve the project objectives safely and within agreed time, cost and performance criteria.*

Martin (2002) identifies budget, time and quality as the three key dimensions to a project. Thus successful projects are completed on time, within the estimated budget, and achieve all of the quality requirements. The job of a project manager and project team (usually public health project workers and often referred to as the steering group) is to keep a balance that enables all of these dimensions to be managed effectively (Martin, 2002), as illustrated in Figure 8.1.

One of the criticisms of this diagram is that the focus is on finance, timescales and outcomes, but a project cannot be achieved without people. The team that carries out all the activities that lead to completing a project are sometimes added in the centre of this diagram (Martin, 2002).

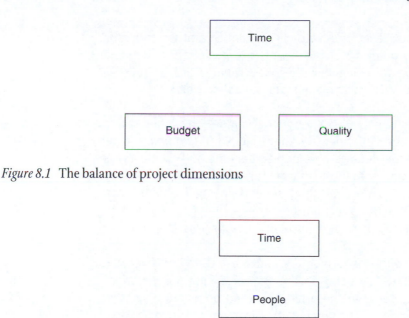

Figure 8.1 The balance of project dimensions

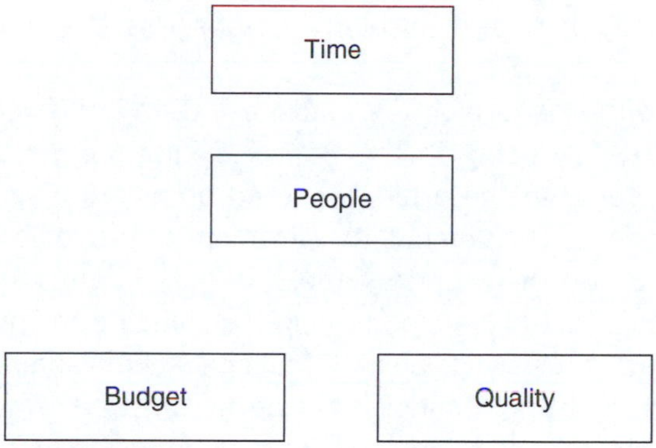

Figure 8.2 The balance of project dimensions – people central

---

ACTIVITY 8.2

Read the case study – 'Getting active' project – and look at Figure 8.2. Think about how any of these key dimensions (timescales, finance, quality) might affect the success of the 'Getting Active' project.

What challenges would you expect Sarah to face if these dimensions are not kept in balance?

Case study: 'Getting Active' project

Sarah, a health improvement manager, set up the 'Getting Active' project, which provides opportunities for people that do little physical activity to take part in physical activity in community settings. It is a complex project involving the trustees of the allotment site, learning support coordinator of the local school, care workers at the day centre, district council health development team, GPs, practice nurses, physiotherapists, other referring health professionals and public health commissioning managers in the local Primary Care Trust (PCT), and Sarah has worked hard to manage this complex project.

The project aim is to encourage people to be more physically active, and funding has been provided for the project for two years, after which time the activities are intended to become self-funding. The budget for the project is made up of a mixture of grants from the local authority community fund and joint commissioning from the local authority and PCT. Sarah is responsible for ensuring that a wide range of activities are available to as many people as possible.

Sarah, together with the project team, knew that not everyone wants to keep active by going to the gym or taking part in sporting activities, and focused the project instead on alternative ways for people to be active. The community allotment is one of a range of activities offered by the project. Others include circuit classes, chair-based exercise, Tai Chi, Chi Do, Qi Gong, line dancing and pilates. The plot at the allotment site has an undercover teaching space, four large growing areas and a polytunnel. It has paths suitable for wheelchair access and raised beds for those who may be less mobile. The activity is linked to healthy eating, where 'cook and taste' sessions are offered. The sessions include recipe ideas that use the produce from the plot.

In establishing the project Sarah, together with the project team, involved local residents and key stakeholders from the outset in designing the project. As a result, the project steering group supported the provision of the wide range of activities offered.

Comment

Each of the dimensions of time, budget and quality are interrelated, and any action affecting any one of the dimensions will impact on both of the others. For example, if the budget is reduced, then there could be an impact on the overall timescale for the activities that are run. Similarly, the quality of the outcomes could be affected if the activities are rushed. In this example, a reduction in budget might mean that fewer activities can be run, or that a smaller range of activities can be funded. The 'Getting Active' project might only be able to offer ten circuit classes, five pilates sessions and one course of Tai Chi, Chi Do and Qi Gong and so on, or only offer circuit classes, Tai Chi and line dancing. This in turn will affect the overall quality of the outcomes from the project. For example, the impact of the project may not be as great as hoped, or the number of participants engaging in activities or continuing in activities may be diminished. Quality in this sense will be seen as the number of participants engaged in the project, or alternatively could be seen as the level of physical activity that is sustained in the longer term.

If Sarah has difficulties in finding staff to run any of the activity sessions offered, this too will have an impact on the overall quality of the project. For example, not being able to offer line dancing to participants as planned would have an impact on the budget and the overall outcomes of the project. In this example, potential participants might be put off attending other activities that have been arranged, and this in turn would impact on the outcomes of the project as a whole.

In summary, if the balance between these three variables (time, budget and quality) is upset then the danger is that the project will fail to meet the expectations of keeping within the agreed budget, finishing on time or producing outcomes of the expected quality.

The other dimension that is clearly important here are the people that are involved in running the project. These include the people who commission the project, those who agree to provide resources as well as those who actually run and take part in the project. For public health projects like this, which need to engage and retain all key stakeholders, the range of key stakeholders is usually wide and the project outcomes multiple. The way in which all these people talk about and behave in relation to the project will be an important element of the project's overall success. Without people, the project cannot be achieved.

The complexity of a project is directly related to its size and scale: the more people involved, the more complicated it becomes. Understanding the key stakeholders and who they are is a crucially important part of the process of defining any public health project. The first step is to consider who the key stakeholders are in the project. In considering this, we need to define stakeholders – these are anyone who has a legitimate interest in the project. They could be your organisation and its directors, your director of public health, local residents, other organisations or sectors, employers and so forth.

In the 'Getting Active' case study there are many different groups of people who are stakeholders and a range of different organisations. Some of the key challenges posed for Sarah are keeping the project on track while managing the varied interests and expectations raised.

Sarah has to ensure that she manages the project in such a way that she attempts to create the perception of successful outcomes from all of the different perspectives held. Keeping all stakeholders engaged in the project is a key challenge for Sarah.

Let's look at the stakeholders in more detail, since gaining their support is crucial to the success of the project. Stakeholders can usually be categorised based on their level of interest and potential influence in the project.

The *project sponsor* is the person or group who sets up the project, authorises the resources and appoints a project manager. The *project team* are the group of people who carry out the tasks and activities to complete the project. There will be a group of stakeholders who have direct control or influence over the outcomes of the project and other who will be directly affected by the project and its outcomes. Each of these stakeholders is likely to have different expectations of the project and use different criteria to gauge its success.

In the 'Getting Active' project, stakeholders can be grouped into the following categories:

- project sponsor;
- project team;
- those who use the facility;
- those who use staff the facility;
- carers;
- local health professionals with an interest but no direct involvement; and
- local residents who may fear additional noise, traffic, disruption, etc.

The life of a project

Regardless of scope or complexity, any project goes through a series of stages during its life. Figure 8.3 illustrates a typical project trajectory, demonstrating the different phases through which a project passes. Looking at the 'Getting Active' project over a two-year timescale, the curve reflects the use of people, financial and material resources during the life cycle of the project. A gradual build-up of activity during which arrangements are made for the project precedes the peak of activity, when the actual project is implemented. The peak is followed immediately by the project's

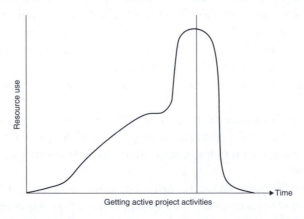

Figure 8.3 The life cycle of a project

conclusion and termination. Each of these phases requires attention to different aspects of the project, and will draw on a range of different tools.

Although all projects differ, they have a series of distinct phases (see Figure 8.4) that they typically pass through: *defining, planning, implementation, closing* and *evaluation* (Martin, 2002). Phase 1, or *Start and Definition*, is completed when the project brief has been written and agreed. Phase 2, *Planning and Specification*, includes all the elements that make up the project plan. Phase 3, *Implementation*, includes all the activities and tasks that achieve the project outcomes. Phase 4, *Closure and Handover*, includes all of the activities and tasks that ensure the project is completed and finished, and Phase 5, *Review and Evaluation*, usually includes evaluation of the outcomes, processes and impact of the project.

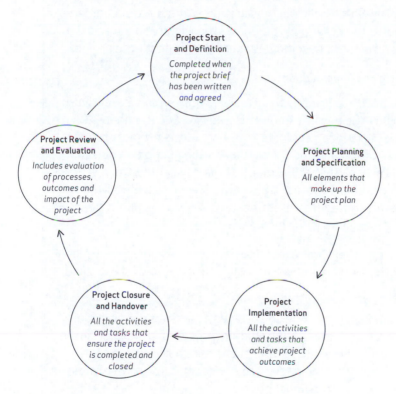

Figure 8.4 The five phases of a project

Source: Adapted from Ewles and Simnett (1999) and Martin (2002)

Seeing a project as having a life cycle with distinct phases enables a focus on what needs to be done in each stage. It also acts as a reminder that the project has a time-limited life and comes to a close. While it is helpful to see these as distinct and discrete stages that are sequentially completed, in reality they are much more likely to be a series of overlapping phases, with the next phase starting before the previous phase is complete.

We will now revisit the 'Getting Active' project case study to illustrate each of these phases.

Case study: 'Getting Active' project revisited

Phase 1: Start and Definition

The project is about increasing levels of physical activity in people who do little physical activity. The intention is to encourage people to take part in activities in community settings rather than in gyms or sporting activities. Funding has been provided for a two-year period, after which it is intended that activities are self-funding.

Turning this into a project brief that can be agreed by all the key stakeholders is a key part of this phase. In this case study the project brief was drawn up by Sarah following discussion with key stakeholders and presented to the steering group. The steering group agreed the project brief and offered to commit resources to support the project.

Phase 2: Planning and Specification

Deciding what needs to be done to increase levels of physical activity in people who do little physical activity is a key part of this phase. This will include talking to local residents, members of the project steering group, trustees of the allotment site, the learning support coordinator of the local school, the care workers at the day centre, the district council health development team, GPs, practice nurses, physiotherapists, other referring health professionals as well as the public health commissioning managers in the local PCT.

Sarah realised that there was a lot to do before it was possible to plan in detail what the 'Getting Active' project could offer and how it could be developed.

Building on a community profile and a needs assessment, Sarah identified a range of activities that could be provided by the project. Discussions with local residents who might take part in these activities enabled Sarah and the wider project team to prioritise those activities that seemed to be most popular.

Growing food in the community allotment, running circuit classes, chair-based exercise, Tai Chi, Chi Do, Qi Gong, line dancing and pilates were all included in the initial project plan. Planning when these different activities would be held was undertaken by a volunteer group of local residents. Scheduling these activities took account of available resources and the need to ensure the quality of all these activities. Clear outcomes for the project were subsequently agreed and a clear schedule of activities developed. The costing for each of these activities was set out in a clear plan, and mechanisms to ensure that the budget was managed effectively were set in place by Sarah.

Phase 3: Implementation

This phase is where Sarah has had the greatest challenge. She has to oversee all of the activities and ensure that the project plan is delivered. Project control and monitoring are the areas where Sarah needs to allocate her time. She constantly monitors the project to check that it is on track against the project plan, and that it is likely to deliver to the specification agreed in the planning phase. Communicating the progress made by the project and identifying key messages for each stakeholder group is an integral part of effective project management. Sarah is keen to keep everyone involved and to ensure that progress is made and communicated to key stakeholders – in particular to the steering group. She arranges for regular review meetings and reports on progress, which can be discussed at the steering group meetings.

Phase 4: Closure and Handover

This phase is planned for from the beginning of the project. When the project ends it is hoped that local residents will continue to take part in the activities offered by the project. Sarah and the project team have been looking at how the project's activities can be sustained from the outset and have regularly sought opportunities for funding from a range of other sources, including working out costs acceptable to local residents. Sarah plans to include this as an agenda item at every steering group meeting.

Phase 5: Review and Evaluation

In this phase Sarah and the project team will need to review whether the project has achieved its goals, and whether it has kept within its planned resources. Sarah is already planning how the evaluation will be done. Sarah is also concerned to ensure that any learning from the project is fed into future projects, and is keeping a record of learning points.

Checklist of key elements in each stage of a project

Phase 1: Project Start and Definition

- Scoping
- Stakeholder analysis and involvement
- Assessing the need – public health evidence*
- Estimating the costs and benefits
- Identifying options*
- Feasibility

* These are not usually included in project definition, but in a public health context they are crucial.

- Feasibility
- Objectives
- Deliverables
- Risk assessment
- Proposal preparation
- Communication.

Phase 2: Planning and Specification

- Time planning
- Scheduling – network diagrams, Gantt charts
- Quality assurance
- Assigning responsibilities
- Risk management
- Communication.

Phase 3: Implementation

- Project control and monitoring
- Time plan
- Resource plan
- Work package specification
- Identified risks
- Communication.

Phase 4: Closure and Handover

- Formal controls for implementing closure – to plan for premature closure
- Procedures for early closure
- Reasons for closure
- Transfer of outcomes and responsibilities
- Learning from project
- Project reporting
- Follow-on actions.

Phase 5: Review and Evaluation

- End of project report
- Lessons learned
- Evaluation – outcomes, processes, impact.

For many public health projects, once the end is reached a new project may start, and multiple projects may be managed simultaneously. Being clear about what needs to be done in which project is a key aspect of the role of a public health project manager. In reality a number of iterations of these project phases take place and each of these phases may be revisited, so this linear representation of a project life cycle may seem a bit simplistic.

Other approaches to project management include the classic six-stage project model, the 7 Questions approach and PRINCE2.

Classic six-stage project model

The classic six-stage project model is useful for more complex projects where a number of phases are carried out simultaneously. This framework emphasises the continuing need for communication throughout the project and has a clear focus on team-building, leading and motivation during the life of the project. This model may be particularly useful for public health projects which are typically complex, involving many different stakeholders and invariably consist of a wide range of concurrent activities. Communicating with stakeholders throughout the life of the project is critical for the success of many public health projects, as is leading, influencing, motivating and networking with others, as indicated in Figure 8.5.

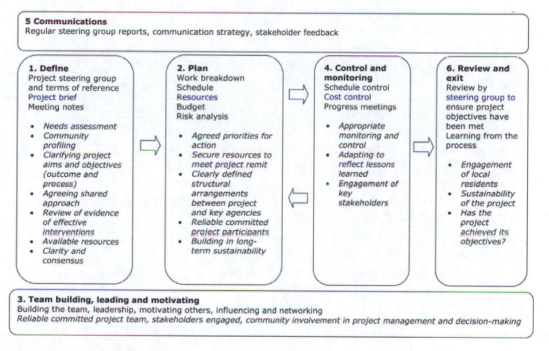

Figure 8.5 Six-stage project-management model

Source: Adapted from Elbeik and Thomas (1998, p14)

The 7 Questions approach

The 7 Questions approach (Martin, 2001) is a practical way to approach a project that has limited implications: that is, fairly low-cost, does not involve large numbers of people or subcontracting with significant budgets. For projects that have wider implications and demand significant accountability, it is generally safer to use a more formal approach and many of the tools and techniques that have been developed for project management (see for example, Field and Keller, 1998; Martin, 2002; Longest, 2004; Martin *et al.*, 2010).

The 7 Questions approach identifies seven key questions that should be asked.

1. What are we trying to do?
2. What is the best way of doing it?
3. What are we going to have to do?
4. In what order should we do things?
5. What resources are we going to need?
6. Review the plan: will it work?
7. Who is going to do what and when?

Using a relatively simple case study example, the next section illustrates the use of the 7 Questions approach.

Case study: Young people's knowledge about sexual health and alcohol

Recently, the Teenage Pregnancy Strategy Partnership board, a multi-agency group consisting of members from local authority, PCTs, charities and third sector organisations, have asked one of the PCTs to undertake a project to explore alcohol and sexual health and the complex links between them for 15–16-year-olds (Year 11) in the local area. The objectives of this project are to explore the prevalence of alcohol misuse and risky sexual behaviour among 15–16-year-olds in order to highlight knowledge, attitudes and behaviours relating to alcohol and sexual health issues, and to inform the commissioning of future services related to alcohol and sexual health so that they are better able to meet the needs of local young people.

Susie, a public health specialist, was asked to manage this project. She has been asked to scope this project in readiness for a sub-group of the Teenage Pregnancy Strategy Partnership board who are due to meet next week. Susie starts by looking at the 7 Questions approach and considering whether this helps to gain a better overview of the project.

What are we trying to do?

This is clear: the aim is to explore alcohol and sexual health and the complex links between them for 15–16-year-olds (Year 11) in the local area.

The objectives are also clear:

- to explore the prevalence of alcohol misuse and risky sexual behaviour among 15–16-year-olds;
- to highlight knowledge, attitudes and behaviours relating to alcohol and sexual health issues;

- to inform the commissioning of future services related to alcohol and sexual health so that they are better able to meet the needs of local young people.

What is the best way of doing it?

Susie considered a range of ways of exploring young people's knowledge, attitudes and behaviours towards sexual health and alcohol, including interviewing young people, holding focus groups and using questionnaires. She decided that developing a questionnaire covering each of the areas in the objectives would provide a good understanding of the self-reported prevalence of alcohol misuse, and the knowledge, attitudes and behaviours relating to alcohol and sexual health, including the complex relationship between them. Focus groups and interviews could be done, but it would take up much more time and require a greater number of staff to carry them out. In addition, it would make sense to do this through schools rather than any other setting.

What are we going to have to do?

Susie made a list of some of the things that would need to be done. Some of these were tasks that she needed to do, while others were tasks that could be delegated or she needed others to do.

- Get buy-in from the Teenage Pregnancy Strategy Partnership board.

- Anticipate any potential risk factors that may emerge.

- Get agreement from schools to take part in the project.

- Gain the co-operation of staff in schools to distribute and collect the questionnaires to and from young people, after they are delivered to the school.

- Gain co-operation from young people to complete the questionnaires.

- Arrange for the information from the questionnaires to be collated and analysed.

- Manage costs to remain within budget.

- Draw up a clear timetable for the project tasks.

- Ensure that progress is monitored and regularly reviewed.

- Develop a clear reporting strategy to inform key stakeholders of plans, progress and outcomes from the project.

- Identify resource implications – data entry, project costs such as printing and distributing questionnaires.

- Calculate any additional costs (over and above those agreed for the project).

In what order should we do things?

Susie set out a first draft of what needs to happen and in what order. Thinking about this made it clear that there were more, and more detailed, tasks which had to be achieved if the project was to be successfully completed. Here are some of the tasks identified by Susie: the more she thought about it, the more she realised there was to do.

- Speak to each of the schools about the project, and get agreement for Year 11 students to participate in the project.
- Develop the questionnaire, get feedback from a small sub-group of the Teenage Pregnancy Strategy Partnership board, and then get the questionnaires printed.
- Agree with each school the process for delivering, distributing and collecting the questionnaires.
- Develop the database ready for data entry and identify who will input the data into the database.
- Take the questionnaires to the schools and support the completion of questionnaires in each of the schools.
- Collect the completed questionnaires from the schools.
- Arrange for the data from the questionnaires to be input into the database.
- Analyse the data gathered and produce a report on the findings.
- Circulate and disseminate the findings to commissioners and present the findings to the Teenage Pregnancy Strategy Partnership board.

Placing each of these activities in order should help Susie to identify any dependent activities. Susie decided that she would draw up a project plan, setting out clearly what needed to be done and when, for approval at the next steering group meeting.

What resources are we going to need?

Looking at resources, Susie could identify the following:

- time for each of the activities identified, and commitment from key stakeholders;
- additional funding to pay for data entry;
- skills to analyse the data gathered;
- funding to cover cost of designing and printing the questionnaires.

ACTIVITY 8.3

What other resources can you identify that might be needed?

Comment

You might have identified the need for some freeing up of staff time, and offering incentives for young people to complete the questionnaires. Susie proposed entering all young people who completed the questionnaires into a draw, with a small prize for the winner.

The next step for Susie was to review whether the ideas that she had noted would be likely to work.

Review the plan: will it work?

Susie realises that it will be important to review the project regularly and monitor progress against the project plan. One observation is that regardless of whatever is planned, unless Susie remains as flexible as she can, it is unlikely to work. It is much more likely that the plan will need to be revised and timelines rescheduled as the project progresses. Building in some contingency just in case the worst happens is a useful consideration.

However, what is really important is that everyone is clear about what they are required to do, and in what revised timeframe. Communication throughout is essential. In public health projects with people based in different organisations, and with many projects running across organisational boundaries, this becomes even more critical.

Who is going to do what and when?

Susie drew up a chart (see Figure 8.6) to make sure that she was clear about what needed doing, when and by whom. She planned to get this agreed at the meeting.

ACTIVITY 8.4

Look at the chart that Susie produced, and consider the relative strengths and weaknesses of this chart.

How might you improve it?

Comment

The chart drawn up by Susie could be viewed as an attempt at scheduling and is often referred to as a Gantt chart. It identifies specific tasks and sets out what needs to be done and when. It also gives some indication of the dependencies that might be involved in the project, or the potential impact that any delay might have on the sequence of tasks. We can see that unless the questionnaires are printed, the young people will not be able to complete them. Because of the way that Susie has identified different work tasks and sequenced them, the impact of a delay is clear.

One improvement that Susie could make to this chart is to identify who is responsible for each of the activities identified. In addition, she could break down each of the identified activities further into more detailed units: for example, the feedback event will need to be planned for, venues will need to be identified, dates and so forth. Susie also might consider adding other information to the chart, such as key milestones to be achieved, project meetings and review dates.

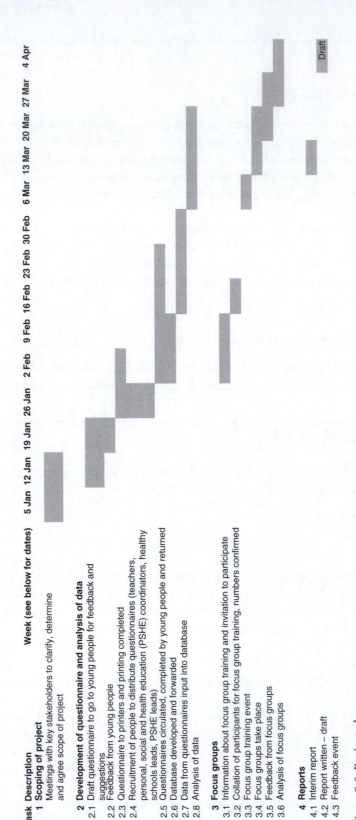

Figure 8.6 Project plan

Delegation was going to be crucial, and Susie knew it was important to ensure that people have delegated authority for each of the activities on the schedule chart, together with clear objectives and delivery dates for their parts of the plan.

It is important to identify activities that cannot start until others have been completed. These activities will determine the overall sequence in which you carry out your project, because you have no option but to do them in that order. Other activities may be less critical, and it may be possible to undertake some of them in parallel. It may be possible for some activities to take place at any time – in which case, you can choose when a suitable point would be to include them.

Other tools that Susie could use include critical path analysis and key events planning (see Martin, 2002, Chapter 8, and Martin *et al.*, 2010, Chapter 18 for some clear examples of these).

PRINCE2

Many public service organisations in the UK use a project management method called PRINCE2 (PRojects IN Controlled Environments), which has been developed and refined over years of use by project managers in many different contexts. PRINCE2 is a process-based method for effective project management. Bentley (2007) sets out its main advantages:

> *PRINCE2 gives:*
>
> – *Controlled management of change by the business in terms of its investment and return on investment*
> – *Active involvement of the users of the final product throughout its development to ensure the business product will meet the functional, environmental, service and management requirements of the users*
> – *More efficient control of development resources.*
>
> (Bentley, 2007, p5)

Areas such as leadership and people management skills are not included in PRINCE2, neither is detailed coverage of project management tools and techniques. Instead, the focus is on the business case, which describes the rationale and business justification for the project (see PRINCE2, nd).

Features of successful projects and some common problems

While there is considerable consensus about the processes, stages and sequence of project management, there is less agreement about how projects may be successfully achieved. Atkinson (1999) notes that the traditional criteria for success (cost, time and quality) are all included in the description of project management. He questions whether this is sufficient, and makes the point that a project may be implemented on time, within cost and meet requested quality parameters, but may not be used by customers or be liked by sponsors. He suggests the need to develop other criteria for success:

> *Customers and users are examples of stakeholders of [information systems] projects*

and the criteria they consider as important for success should also be included in assessing a project.

(Atkinson, 1999, p340)

Within the context of public health, any project that has failed to engage key stakeholders is unlikely to be successful. Identifying the criteria considered by stakeholders to be important for success needs to be included.

In reviewing a large number of projects, Elbeik and Thomas (1998) found ten key factors identified by managers in multinational organisations that are perceived to be critical to the success of a project:

1. clearly defined objectives;

2. good planning and control;

3. a good-quality project manager;

4. good management support;

5. sufficient time and resource;

6. commitment by all;

7. high user involvement;

8. good communications;

9. good project organisation and structure;

10. the ability to stop a project.

ACTIVITY 8.5

Think about a project in which you have been involved.

How many of these factors are present?

What problems might be experienced in a project?

What does this suggest about the common problems that projects might experience?

Comment

Common problems identified include the project team being unsure of the project objectives and lack of clarity about the project deliverables. Sometimes at the end of a project, the objectives have been only partially achieved. The planned schedule might have run late, and the budget might have been exceeded. Those who were expected to make use of the project outcomes may have not have understood, liked or wanted to use them. Another problem that is often identified too late is the project that has not been stopped effectively, and which has become more like a routine activity for the participants. All projects have an endpoint: it is important that a project is brought to a close. Developing plans for the sustainability of a project may lead to new projects, or the project may develop into a programme which, as stated at the beginning of this chapter, is different from a project.

Chapter summary

In this chapter we began by considering what distinguishes a project from a programme or the normal day-to-day tasks of managing. The main features of a project and a number of different stages in the project life cycle were identified. Some key tools and techniques to manage these different stages were introduced. The importance of defining the scope of a public health project and working with key stakeholders, running and keeping the project on track, knowing when to hand the project over and ensuring that the project is evaluated and reported on, were emphasised.

The complexity of many public health and health promotion projects makes project management increasingly important. Effective project management ensures that the project will achieve its intended outcomes. The project manager's role in leading, communicating the vision of the project outcome and gaining support from key stakeholders is crucial to the effectiveness of any project. The classic six-stage project management model and the 7 Questions approach were introduced, and the 7 Questions approach applied to a simple case study in order to demonstrate how this may be used effectively to manage less complex projects. PRINCE2 was introduced as a method used to manage projects in the public sector in the UK. Finally, the key features of successful projects and some common problems were considered.

GOING FURTHER

Field, M and Keller, L (1998) *Project Management*. London: Open University/Thomson Learning.
This book provides a clear overview of project management, covering all the basic principles. It is designed to equip the reader with the knowledge and techniques to manage projects successfully. All stages of managing a project are covered, and the book is intended for people managing a project in all kinds of organisations.

Martin V (2002) *Managing Projects in Health and Social Care*. Abingdon: Routledge.
This title provides a practical overview and clear examples of managing projects in health and social care contexts. See Chapter 8 for examples of critical path analysis.

Martin, V, Charlesworth, J and Henderson, E (2010) *Managing in Health and Social Care* (2nd edn). Abingdon: Routledge.
Chapter 18 introduces a range of techniques in planning and managing projects in the context of health and social care, including clear examples of critical path analysis.

PRINCE2
http://webarchive.nationalarchives.gov.uk/20110822131357/http:// www.ogc.gov.uk/methods_prince_2.asp
The official site for PRINCE2, which provides detailed information on PRINCE2, training and background development.

chapter 9

Leading and Managing Change
Vicki Taylor

Meeting the Public Health Competences

This chapter will help you to evidence the following competences for public health (Public Health Skills and Career Framework):

- Level 5(4) Contribute effectively to change within own area of work;
- Level 5(g) Awareness of drivers and levers of change relevant to own area of work;
- Level 6(4) Contribute effectively to change and developments within own area of work;
- Level 6(g) Knowledge of change management theories and their application;
- Level 6(h) Knowledge of drivers and levers of change in own area of work;
- Level 7(4) Lead and influence change in own area of work;
- Level 7(g) Knowledge of frameworks for managing change;
- Level 8(5) Lead change in a complex environment, handling uncertainty, the unexpected and conflicts appropriately;
- Level 8(g) Understanding of frameworks for managing change.

This chapter will also assist you in demonstrating the following National Occupational Standards for public health:

- Lead change (M&L_C4);
- Plan change (M&L_C5);
- Implement change (M&L_C6).

In addition, this chapter will be useful in demonstrating Standard 10d of the Public Health Practitioner Standards:

Standard 10. Support the implementation of policies and strategies to improve health and wellbeing outcomes – demonstrating:

d. the ability to prioritise and manage projects and/or services in own area of work.

Overview

This chapter will help you to develop your thinking about managing change and, in particular, managing change to improve health. In this chapter we will explore some of the theory relating to change management and consider the implications for public health and health promotion. Key themes in change management are introduced and the conceptual frameworks used in thinking about managing change are explored. Kotter's eight-steps framework for managing change is described in order to help identify ways to manage change more effectively, and a number of useful tools that can be used in managing change are introduced. Finally, we will consider some key features of successful change management approaches and look at some of the common problems experienced in managing change.

The activities in this chapter will focus on:

- developing clarity about the nature of change;
- considering key drivers for change;
- appreciating the driving and restraining forces for change;
- understanding the different phases in the change process;
- using an eight-step model to plan for and implement change;
- utilising tools such as commitment planning, stakeholder analysis and force-field analysis which can be used in managing public health change projects;
- exploring some commonly used strategic approaches to change and approaches to managing resistance to change.

After reading this chapter you will be able to:

- identify some of the drivers for change;
- identify the main features of managing change;
- understand the different stages in change management;
- understand and use some of the main change management tools and techniques;
- develop a critical awareness of the importance of people in change management and, in particular, stakeholders.

Why consider change management?

Public health and health promotion are essentially about achieving change in order to improve health. Change was a central element of the World Health Organization (WHO) programme on health promotion (WHO, 1984; Green and Tones, 2010) when it was first established, and it remains so today. Thus action for health improvement requires a focus on, and skills in, managing change.

Public health practitioners are involved in setting up, planning, implementing and managing change across a wide range of different agencies, initiatives, projects and programmes. Change is at the heart of public health and health promotion. It could be argued that the key purpose of public health and health promotion is to create change in order to achieve improvements in health. Creating public health policy, acting as an advocate for specific communities and groups, and using change initiatives to increase and empower communities, are activities central to the achievement of improvement in health. Such change is at the social, environmental and political levels as well as at the individual level.

Despite the importance of change management in achieving health improvement, there has been little attention paid in the health promotion and public health literature to change management theory and skills, or to the development of skills to manage and produce change. As Dooris and Hunter (2007, p111) note, there is a proliferation of literature associated with change management; however, very little of this focuses on change in relation to pubic health and health promotion. Rather, attention has focused on the theoretical aspects of behaviour change, models and frameworks to explain and help understand how and why individuals change their behaviour, and how these can be used as tools in promoting health.

More recently, the use of marketing techniques to achieve change, referred to as social marketing, have received attention. While these are legitimate areas of focus, organisational change and managing such processes in order to increase health outcomes has received little attention by comparison. In their review of managing change in the NHS, Iles and Sutherland draw attention to the need for staff to become *more skilled in handling change in a complex environment with multiple stakeholders, conflicting objectives and considerable constraints* (2001, p19). Senior (2002) observes that successful change management is a highly required skill. Public health practitioners who work both within and across organisations and partnerships, and manage multiple stakeholders, are in particular need of developing skills to facilitate change.

Dooris and Hunter claim that *public health practitioners and others engaged in promoting health are poorly equipped to function in a way that is likely to bring about significant improvements in health* (2007, p110). They go on to suggest that organisational development and change management are vital tools in achieving improvements in health.

The nature of change

The literature on change management and organisational change is large and not easy to access (Iles and Sutherland, 2001), and there is a sense that much of what exists is contradictory or not particularly practical. By (2005) provides a critical review of organisational change management, concluding that there appears to be no common agreement on a framework for the successful management of organisational change despite the consensus that the pace of change has never been greater and that change, whether triggered by internal or external factors, *comes in all shapes, forms and sizes* (2005, p370).

There is considerable debate within the literature on the nature of change and whether it is continuous, incremental, discontinuous or a combination of all of these. Grundy defines discontinuous change as change *which is marked by rapid shifts in either strategy, structure or culture, or in all three* (1993, p26). Others refer to this as radical or revolutionary change, as it is often associated with fundamental change (Alvesson and Willmott, 2001). Nelson suggests that often there are periods of incremental change crammed in between *more violent periods of (discontinuous) change* (2003, p18).

Within the public health context it would seem that current organisational change in England (i.e. the shift of public health from the NHS to local government, as mentioned previously in this book) triggered by external political policy, as set out in the White Paper on public health (Department of Health, 2010b), could be described as discontinuous. Interestingly, the literature suggests that this approach is an inefficient one, and that discontinuous change can lead to a cyclical process of *defensive behaviour, complacency, inward focus, and routines, which again creates situations where major reform is frequently required* (By, 2005, p372). Furthermore, it is suggested that the benefits from such change do not last.

Whether change is planned or emergent is another ongoing theme in the literature. The current consensus seems to be that the idea of planned change is outmoded and at best too simplistic, given the need for organisations to respond constantly to their external environment. Three criticisms are levelled at the notion of planned change (By, 2005, p374). First, it is argued that planned change is not relevant to situations requiring rapid and transformational change. Second, the underlying assumptions of planned change – that an organisation can move from one state to another stable state – are argued as being irrelevant in the context of an increasingly unstable external environment. Third, it is suggested that *the approach of planned change ignores situations where more directive approaches are required* (By, 2005, p374). By (2005) suggests that such criticism has led to increased support for an emergent approach to organisational change, where change is seen as being driven from the 'bottom-up'. As By notes, instead of pre-planned steps to be followed, an emergent approach to change is focused more on developing *change readiness and facilitating for change* (2005, p375). This seems to have much in common with working for health improvement. It is an approach that is focused on developing change management skills and creating change agents at all levels, and across and within organisations involved in promoting and improving health.

Drivers for change

In thinking about change and change management, it is useful to begin by considering some of the drivers of change. Group and professional norms can be an important force in resisting and/or driving change. From a public health and health promotion perspective, the key drivers are the desire to improve the public's health and wellbeing. Changes are usually required to ensure that the health potential of all citizens is maximised. In the UK (and globally) it is clear that there are wide disparities in the health status of those with the poorest health and those with the best health. Furthermore, much of this disparity can be attributed to unequal opportunities or inequalities in health. Inequalities in health exist in relation to social class, geographic location, gender, ethnicity and income (Dahlgren and Whitehead, 1991; Acheson, 1998; Sacker *et al.*, 2000; Dorling *et al.*, 2007; Graham and Kelly, 2004; Marmot, 2007, 2010; Aldridge *et al.*, 2011) that require action, which in turn requires change of some kind. Whether this action is at an individual level, or more focused on social action, the drivers are similar. Reducing inequalities in health and maximising health gain for all are two key drivers. These are underpinned by a commitment to equity and social justice. Healthy public policy was a key element of the WHO view of health promotion, which viewed it as central to the transformation (and therefore change) of society in order to improve health (Douglas *et al.*, 2007).

Other drivers for change include political imperatives, policy initiatives such as the recent decision to locate public health within local government, a desire by decision-makers for wholesale change rather than incremental evolution, an ever-changing policy context, and financial imperatives such as cost pressures. Population and democratic drivers for change also may act as a big influence, together with environmental considerations.

ACTIVITY 9.1

Consider your own work or your own organisation.

What are the key drivers for change?

How do these affect the work that you do?

How could you use these drivers to help you to improve health?

To what extent do these drivers hinder you in improving health?

Are the drivers for organisational change different to those drivers for change for health improvement? If so, how?

Comment

Recent drivers for change in public health organisations include:

- political direction;
- legislation;
- regulation;
- reduction of inequalities in health; and
- the shift to partnership with a wider commercial market.

You may have focused on general financial and global pressures, or indeed identified more specific financial drivers, such as the nature of short-term funding and the need to review and scale down activity or to change what is done. Wanless (2002, 2004), for example, notes that continuing to do the same thing in the same way, that is, treating illness, will inevitably lead to bankruptcy. Newly-published evidence of effectiveness and policy guidance from the National Institute for Clinical Excellent (NICE) or the Department of Health are key drivers for change within public health.

Many of these drivers are welcome and are about improving the effectiveness of health promotion and developing successful public health projects, but often they can feel imposed and appear to be yet another initiative that is being driven 'top-down'. To what extent is action from the grass roots a driver for change? This was one of the central values of health promotion and strengthened at the Second

---

International Conference on Health Promotion in Adelaide (WHO, 1988), where local community action was viewed as a major driving force.

You may have noticed that many of these drivers share a common attribute: they are all external to the organisation. It is not a requirement that drivers are external to the organisation, but given the continually changing external environment, it is not surprising that many drivers are. You might find it useful to refer to Chapter 3, where the PESTLE analysis was introduced. Do any of the influences you identified in Activity 3.4 recur in your response to Activity 9.1?

Force-field analysis: a tool for assessing readiness for change

Reviewing the drivers for change, and their counteracting resistors or forces against change, can be useful in two ways. First, it can be used to assess the prospects for change, helping to form a view on the feasibility of change and the likelihood of its success. Second, it can be useful as a tool to identify ways to shift the balance in favour of change. Lewin (1951) developed a simple tool to analyse drivers (or driving forces) and resistors (or restraining forces). Lewin suggested that all the forces that may help drive change should be identified, and then to assess how 'big' each driver is. These are represented on one side (or top) of a diagram as arrows pushing in the direction of change, with the length and thickness of each arrow representing the strength of the force. Identifying the restraining forces and representing these on the other side (or bottom) of the diagram is the next step (as in Figure 9.1).

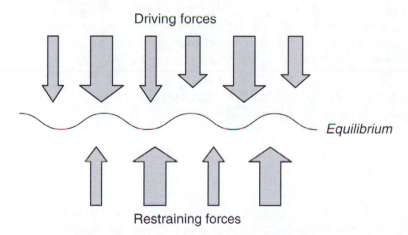

Figure 9.1 A force-field analysis

Source: Adapted from Lewin (1951)

When the forces pushing in one direction exceed those pushing in the opposite direction, the existing equilibrium is changed. Lewin (1951) asserted that increasing the driving forces is more likely to result in an increase in the resisting forces, such that the current equilibrium is not changed but maintained under increased tension. He suggested that reducing resisting forces was preferable to attempts to increase driving forces, as this results in greater movement towards the desired state without increasing tension. Criticisms of Lewin's force-field analysis are that the model is too simplistic, given the complexity of organisations; also, it has been suggested that there may be no such thing as equilibrium. However, Lewin's force field analysis remains a useful tool to diagnose and plan interventions.

Case study: Considering a change in ways of working with the community

Rose has been working as a public health improvement worker for three years. So far she has achieved a lot since taking up her post, including developing some very good women's health networks and supporting a number of women's health forums to publicise breast and cervical screening programmes in the area. She meets regularly with more than 20 women's groups, and is asked to give presentations and one-to-one sessions, all of which are enjoyable and fulfilling.

However, this is very time-consuming, and currently she is exploring the possibility of changing the way that she works with the community so that she can develop community group members to provide outreach to encourage women to take up the offer of breast and cervical screening, and to give presentations and one-to-one sessions with women.

Using a force-field analysis, Rose can represent the current situation as a horizontal line. The driving forces (i.e. those forces or reasons that are supportive of change) can be represented as downward-pointing arrows that are seeking to push the line. The restraining forces (i.e. those forces or reasons that are likely to resist change) can then be represented by upward-pointing arrows that are supporting the line (the current situation) and seeking to keep it where it is. Using this completed diagram she can see how feasible this proposed change is, and can easily identify ways to minimise the resistors.

ACTIVITY 9.2

Think of a public health initiative, project or change you would like to implement, or in which you are currently involved. It can be a simple or more complex change. Identify the forces for change, and then identify the likely resistance to change.

Now construct a diagram like Figure 9.1 to illustrate the forces that are supportive of the change (the driving forces), and those forces that are likely to be resistant (the restraining forces).

How might the restraining forces be minimised?

Can you identify ways to shift the balance between the drivers and resistors in favour of change?

Comment

In the case study Rose identified management pressure to be more cost-effective and the need to demonstrate a wider coverage of community groups in the area as key drivers for change. Both of these drivers were strong and having a direct impact on Rose's workload. An expectation of her to work with, and develop ways of working with, communities in the west of the area was a further key driver. In addition, the shifting of resources to a more deprived neighbourhood and a policy directive to reduce inequalities in health were important drivers.

The resistors that Rose identified were the need to develop the skills and confidence of some of the women's health group members, and to support the transition. However, on the positive side, two women had suggested already that they could take on some outreach work as part of their community development role funded by the council. Another potential restraining force might be the perception that this was a cost-cutting exercise, and that women's health work was being cut. She concluded that on balance, the drivers far outweighed the resistors.

Using the force field analysis, Rose was able to identify ways to minimise the resistors. She reasoned that provided that she could get agreement for some development and training sessions for at least four of the women's health group members, and provide some initial support during the transition, most likely she would be able to implement these changes. These actions would minimise the impact of the restraining forces. She also identified the need to work with community networks to develop new networks in the west of the area, in order to develop community-based initiatives to reduce inequalities in health.

Phases in the change process

Lewin (1951) identified three phases in the change process: unfreezing, changing and refreezing. The first phase, unfreezing, is often viewed as critical and has been referred to as *preparing the ground* (Pettigrew and Whipp, 1993, p6). Creating the climate for change is an important part of this phase. Getting people to accept the need for change and preparing them for it is a key part of this phase. The second phase is focused on implementing and undergoing the change and all that this entails. Often this is the most difficult phase, as people confront the change and begin to realise the implications for themselves and the organisation. The third phase, refreezing, involves embedding and consolidating the change. The importance of this phase is often overlooked; however, it is crucial, as it is concerned with reinforcing the change and ensuring that this becomes the new norm.

Building on Lewin's phases, Bullock and Batten (1985) developed a four-phase model. They suggest that the first phase is 'exploration', which determines whether there is a need for change. The second phase is 'planning', which involves understanding the nature of the problem, developing objectives for the change and choosing the approach to change. During this stage key stakeholders are identified, and the processes to involve them introduced. The third phase, 'action', is the implementation stage: during this stage, monitoring is critical. The fourth phase is 'integration'. It is at this point that the change is fully integrated and embedded, and evaluation to look at the effectiveness of the change can begin. Table 9.1 compares Lewin and Bullock and Batten's three-phase and four-phase models.

Table 9.1 A comparison of Lewin's three-stage model and Bullock and Batten's four-phase model

Lewin	Bullock and Batten
Unfreezing	Exploration
	Planning
Changing	Action
Refreezing or consolidating	Integration

Case study: Changing public health in England

In the current context, moving public health from the NHS to local government requires a shift in thinking about where public health sits. In November 2010 the English government published a new strategy for public health in a White Paper, *Healthy Lives, Healthy People: Our Strategy for Public Health in England* (Department of Health, 2010b). This White Paper set the scene for the government's intention to create a new public health system in England. The reforms include the development of a new executive agency – Public Health England – and subject to parliamentary agreement, the transition of public health from the NHS to local government. Through this White Paper, the government began the process of creating the climate for change and preparing the ground for what could be viewed as radical change.

In July 2011, *Healthy Lives, Healthy People White Paper: Update and Way Forward* (Department of Health, 2011a) was published, which is a summary of responses to *Healthy Lives, Healthy People: Our Strategy for Public Health in England*. Other publications such as *Healthy Lives, Healthy People: Consultation on the Funding and Commissioning Routes for Public Health* (Department of Health, 2011b) and *Healthy Lives, Healthy People: Transparency In Outcomes – Proposals for a Public Health Outcomes Framework* (Department of Health, 2011c) were published in the same month. All of these publications, and the consultations with key stakeholders associated with these documents, can be viewed as the move into the next phase: the implementation phase. More details of the design of the new public health system, specifically the role and responsibilities of local government in public health, the operating model for the new executive agency Public Health England and an overview of how the whole system will work, have now been published. A clear timetable has been produced and more detailed implications set out. A series of factsheets have been produced *to further inform stakeholders and staff involved in the new public health system so that the reforms can be implemented effectively* (Department of Health, 2011d).

At the time of writing we are still in the early part of Lewin's second phase. It will be interesting to see how these changes are consolidated and embedded – or, to paraphrase Bullock and Batten, how these changes are 'integrated'. The case study below looks at a much less complex change.

ACTIVITY 9.3

Read the following case study, 'Changing the health promotion resource loan system', and look at Table 9.1. Think about whether and how each of Lewin and Bullock and Batten's key phases are undertaken in the case study.

What challenges would you expect Grace to face in each of these phases?

How might thinking about each of these phases help to prepare you to manage the changes that you face?

Case study: Changing the health promotion resource loan system

Grace was responsible for the health promotion resource centre with a team of 15 staff, divided between two buildings. For some time she had been reviewing the location of the resources and the way that the loan system operated. It was costly in terms of staff time, and seemed rather cumbersome and out-of-date, requiring lengthy booking in and booking out procedures. In addition, the resources were in a separate building. Over a period of three months Grace regularly held discussions with the team on the need for a new system, and explored the team members' views on the existing location.

Subsequently, the director of public health agreed that a new system should be found, and proposed that it would be cost-effective to move the resources into the same building as the rest of the team. Grace was asked to plan and implement the changes. First, she reviewed possible library systems and visited other health promotion resource units and libraries. She discussed possible options with key stakeholders, including the staff in her team and users of the health promotion resource library. She sought their views, concerns and expectations. She identified a number of potential solutions and devised a system for booking resources that could be managed by one of the administrators. She also worked with the rest of the team to develop some ideas on how the resources could be moved into the existing space. The decision to move the resources into the largest room, and for staff to be grouped together in an open plan environment, was supported by all.

Grace worked together with the team to consider the implications of this, and developed some new ways of working that included a booking system for the remaining office, so that meetings could take place there rather than in the open plan area.

When the new resource centre had been established and the office moves had taken place, Grace reviewed and monitored the changes. It became clear that the booking system for resources was proving to be a great success. All of the team used the new system to book resources in and out. Grace was amazed how much greater involvement there was.

Comment

In raising the location and running of the existing service with all the team members, Grace in effect began the unfreezing phase. She raised the possibility of alternatives and presented a way of thinking about the service differently. By the time that the director of public health proposed co-locating the health promotion resource loan system into the same building as the rest of the department, most members of the team were already open to new ideas. This led to a relatively smooth implementation phase. Once the change had been integrated and embedded, it was monitored, and an evaluation to look at the effectiveness of the change identified a number of initial teething problems. These were discussed with all the team members so that there was greater ownership of the change. This in turn supported the refreezing phase and consolidation of the change.

Kanter *et al.* (1992, p16) identify three different roles in the change process:

1. *change strategists* – initiators of the change process;
2. *change implementers* – who co-ordinate and bring about the change;
3. *change recipients* – who are affected by the change.

In the case study example above, we can see that Grace is both a change strategist and change implementer. The members of the team could be seen as both change recipients and change implementers. The director of public health appears to be a change strategist. Kanter *et al.* suggest that although these roles are distinct, individuals may inhabit more than one of them at any given time in the change process.

Now, let's turn to look at the process of change in more detail – in particular, Kotter's eight-step model.

The process of change: Kotter's eight-step model

Mento *et al.* (2002) identify three models of change management which have stood as exemplars within the change management literature. These include Kotter's eight-step model, Jick's tactical ten-step model for implementing change, and General Electric's seven-step change acceleration process model. Here we will focus on Kotter's eight-step model. In his influential paper, Kotter (1995, p59) reports that in his study of more than 100 companies, the vast majority of change efforts were unsuccessful. Two key lessons identified by Kotter are that each step or phase needs to be worked through in order for change to be successful, and that mistakes in any phase will have an impact on the overall change process. Kotter identified eight mistakes that are commonly made by organisations when planning for and implementing change, which led to the development of an eight-step change model as summarised in Figure 9.2.

Step 1: Establish a sense of urgency

This step involves inspiring and motivating people to support the change and to actively create a sense of speed. Establishing the need for change is an important part of this step, and both internal and external factors, such as policy directives or the sudden departure of a member of staff, may be important triggers for change. Kotter suggests that this stage is crucial, and that unless around 75 per cent of an organisation's management is convinced that change is essential, then it is unlikely to be successful.

Step 2: Form a powerful guiding coalition

In this stage, the focus is on getting people in place with the right emotional commitment, and the right mix of skills and levels to drive the change process. The leadership coalition grows as time progresses, and a snowballing effect can be seen. Kotter

(1995, p62) found that successful organisational transformations had a powerful guiding coalition, frequently made up of staff outside of the normal hierarchy that worked well together, had strong leadership and acted as a powerful force for change. Developing this guiding coalition is key to successful change, as well as ensuring that the coalition is sufficiently powerful to overcome any opposition and maintain progress.

Step 3: Create a vision

Creating a vision to direct the change and developing strategies to achieve that vision were identified by Kotter as being key requirements for successful change efforts, but are often lacking. The ability to create a clear vision and to get others to share and, indeed, to shape it, should not be underestimated. Kotter sets out a useful rule of thumb for this step: if the vision cannot be communicated *in five minutes or less* and *get a reaction that signifies both understanding and interest* (1995, p63), then further work is needed.

Step 4: Communicate the vision

In this step, involving as many people as possible, communicating the new vision and strategy and ensuring that this vision is understandable to key stakeholders, is paramount. Winning hearts and minds is an integral element of this step and a further opportunity to gain commitment to the change process. This will be especially important where there are short-term sacrifices (Kotter, 1995, p63). The phrase 'walking the talk' is imperative in this stage of the change process, as communication is seen both through words and actions.

Step 5: Empower others to act on the vision

In this step, removing obstacles, enabling constructive feedback and support from leaders and encouraging creativity in taking the change forward are all central. Inevitably, there will be some employees (and indeed other stakeholders) who do not support the change and might actively resist it. As the change progresses in time, an increasing number of people are involved, and so organisations that support employees to develop new ideas and ways of working that reflect the vision need to be supported and empowered to do this.

Step 6: Planning and creating short-term wins

Setting achievable aims and recognising and rewarding employees involved in the change is the focus of this step. Providing compelling evidence of success and quick wins that demonstrate some expected results are often necessary at this stage in order to keep the change initiative going (Kotter states that this might be around 12–24 months in the change process). A failure to do this can lead to people giving up or joining those who are resisting the change. In addition, commitment to producing short-term wins can help keep up the urgency level (Kotter, 1995, p66).

Step 7: Consolidate improvements and continue change

Using increased credibility and changing systems, structures and policies to fit the vision is central to this step of the change process. Reinvigorating the change and supporting change agents to continue the process are activities that need to be continued, in some cases for as long as ten years. One of the biggest problems is that all too often, organisations declare successful change too early, and within two years or so the changes that have been achieved slowly disappear (Kotter, 1995, p66).

Step 8: Institutionalise new approaches

This final stage involves reinforcing successful change and rooting changes in the social norms and shared values of the organisation: what Kotter refers to as *anchoring changes in the organisation's culture* (1995, p67). Modelling new behaviours and attitudes is important, as is succession planning and embedding the values and ways of working in the next generation of management. This stage is the one that is often omitted, as the importance of cultural change and the length of time that it takes may be easily overlooked (see Chapter 3 for a more detailed discussion of organisational culture).

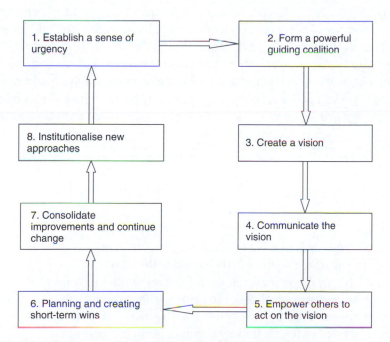

Figure 9.2 An eight-step model for planning and managing change

Source: Adapted from Kotter (1995)

ACTIVITY 9.4

Think of a public health initiative, project or change in which you are currently involved, or of which you have experience. Consider (or find out, if you do not know) how this initiative was planned for, and how the changes were implemented.

Now consider each of the steps in Kotter's eight-step model.

Can you identify whether and how any of these steps were built into the change process? If not, what needs to be done to move through each of these steps successfully?

How can you plan for each step?

What are the implications for your own role as a public health practitioner?

Comment

You may have found it difficult to recognise all of these steps, as in many cases the change is unplanned and there is no consideration of any framework to guide the change initiative or project. Even when there is clear planning and a framework such as Kotter's eight-step model is used, it is unsurprising that it can be difficult to identify each of the steps in practice. Often the process is not linear, and different steps may be revisited or merge together: rarely is the implementation of change straightforward. This particularly true for the complex change initiatives that we are usually concerned with in public health and health promotion. Initiatives that aim to improve health or reduce inequalities in health are complicated further, because they often need to be implemented across different organisations and within complex environments and contexts. This complexity makes the use of frameworks to plan for and consider how to manage and implement change all the more vital. Two other tools, stakeholder analysis and commitment planning, are valuable in identifying those who need to be influenced or involved in the change process and in assessing their commitment to the proposed initiatives.

Stakeholder analysis

A technique called stakeholder analysis is widely used in managing change. It consists of identifying the key stakeholders, and then ranking them on two dimensions: power and interest. Power measures the influence that they have over the change project, and the degree to which they can help to achieve or block the desired change. Interest measures the level of interest that they have in the change and, if they are affected by that change, their likely alignment with it. These can be plotted in one of the four quadrants in the Stakeholder Influence map (Figure 9.3).

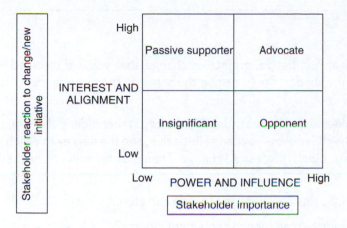

Figure 9.3 Stakeholder influence map

Different strategies are then used, depending on which quadrant the stakeholders are placed in (see Figure 9.4).

Stakeholders with high power and interests aligned with the change initiative are the people who need to be fully engaged and brought on board. Actively influencing these stakeholders and working closely with them is a priority.

Those with high alignment and interest but low power and influence need to be kept informed. When organised, they may form the basis of an interest group which can lobby for change. Increasing the power or influence of these stakeholders can be a useful strategy to gain increased support for an initiative. This is a legitimate activity and is at the core of public health advocacy work.

Those with high power but low interest need to be kept satisfied and, if possible, influenced to become supporters for the proposed change. Stakeholders in the bottom left-hand quadrant with low alignment and interest and low power and influence should be monitored.

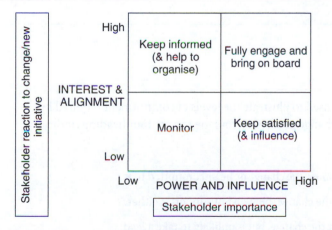

Figure 9.4 Strategies for working with stakeholders (based on their power and influence and interest in and alignment with the proposed change)

ACTIVITY 9.5

Think of a public health initiative, project or change that you are involved with, or one that you want to undertake (it can be the same as the one you identified in Activity 9.2 or 9.4).

Carry out a stakeholder analysis. First, identify the key stakeholders, then consider the influence that they have over the change initiative, and the degree to which they can help to achieve or block the desired change. Then plot them in one of the four quadrants.

What implications does this analysis have for the initiative?

How might this help you to plan for and implement change?

What actions would you suggest, based on your stakeholder analysis?

Comment

In carrying out a stakeholder analysis, it is likely that you will have identified a need for more information, or a need to know more about some of the stakeholders that you identified. For example, you might have identified a need to find out what information they want from you and how they would like that information provided. Also, you may want to gauge the opinion of a specific stakeholder of both your work and the public health project that you are seeking to implement. You may be interested to find out what is likely to influence their views, or how you might gain their backing. If they are unlikely to be supportive, you may want to consider (or find out) what will win them around to support this project; alternatively, if you suspect that they are unlikely to support the initiative, how you will manage their opposition. It is also worth considering those who they might influence and how you will manage this. Your stakeholder analysis should help you to identify those stakeholders on whom you need to focus most of your energy and attention.

Commitment planning

A commitment plan can be used to illustrate the levels of commitment required by different stakeholders in a change process. Across the top are four headings indicating levels of commitment:

1. *Opposed* – likely to oppose the change or be uncommitted to it.

2. *Let* – will not oppose the change, but will not support it either.

3. *Support* – will support the change, but is unlikely to take a lead.

4. *Lead* – will lead the change process and make it happen.

Key stakeholders (individuals or groups) affected by a change are then listed down one side: this helps to determine how committed they are to the intended change. In the columns to the right, an X is placed in the column representing their current level of commitment. Next, an O is placed in the column representing the level of commitment needed if the change is likely to be achieved. The difference between the two positions is an indication of the work to be done in order to build the support needed to progress the change. It can help you to determine where to focus your efforts, and to indicate who needs to be committed to the change initiative.

Table 9.2 Commitment plan

Individuals	*Opposed*	*Let*	*Support*	*Lead*
1.	X		O	
2.		X	O	
3.		X		X
4.				XO
5.		XO		

ACTIVITY 9.6

Think of a public health initiative, project or change you are involved with, have already undertaken or want to undertake (it can be the same as the one you identified in Activity 9.2 or 9.4). Draw a commitment plan.

What implications does this plan have for the change project?

How might this help you to plan for and implement change?

What are the key learning points from this consideration?

Comment

In carrying out this activity, it is likely that you will have identified a number of stakeholders who were not committed to the change. However, while there are some key stakeholders whose support is critical, commitment will not be needed from all stakeholders, and commitment planning can help you distinguish between them. Used in conjunction with force-field and stakeholder analyses, a commitment plan can help you to be more precise about the extent to which commitment is necessary.

What's the evidence?

Thurley and Wirdenius (1973) identified five commonly used strategic approaches to change (directive, expert, negotiated, educative and participative), which they categorised depending on the degree to which the change was imposed. These different approaches are not mutually exclusive, and can be used in conjunction with one another. A summary of the key characteristics of each of these approaches follows.

Directive strategies

Change is usually imposed through management authority and follows a plan set out by management. There is little involvement of other people in the change process. A directive approach has the advantage that it can be carried out quickly; however, the main disadvantage is that it does not take any account of the views or feelings of those affected by the change. One of the consequences of not involving those affected is that this can increase the likelihood of resistance, which in turn can reduce the speed of the change and potentially undermine it. In order to be effective, directive strategies require strong personal and position power, relevant information and an ability to manage opposition and resistance. Directive approaches can be often found in times of crisis and 'turnaround' situations.

Expert strategies

This approach is appropriate when the change is driven by a technical problem that requires a solution by experts. Specialist skills and expertise, from both inside and outside the organisation, are used to bring about the change. The central focus of an expert approach to change is in ensuring that the best technical solution to the problem requiring change is both found and implemented. There is little involvement or consideration of those affected by the change. The advantages of expert strategies are that they bring in expertise, which can be used to consider the change problem in more detail, and the implementation of change is relatively quick. A potential disadvantage is that the proposed solution (and therefore the proposed changes) may not be one that is shared by the people that the problem affects, which in turn may lead to resistance to the change.

Negotiated strategies

Negotiated strategies involve some bargaining about the changes. They demonstrate both an awareness of, and willingness to, discuss the changes, and enable those affected by the change to have some say in it. This can be an important strategy when buy-in is needed, and as an approach it can be useful in reducing resistance to change. The disadvantage is that implementation may take a little longer and outcomes can be less easily predicted.

Educative strategies

This approach has an underpinning assumption that one needs people to share similar values and beliefs if one is to bring about successful change. The emphasis of an educative strategy is to win hearts and minds through a mixture of activities such as persuasion, education, training and selection. The advantage of this approach, when successful, is that people will be positively committed to the change. A possible disadvantage is that it can take much longer than the previous approaches.

Participative strategies

This approach to change has as an underlying assumption that people will not be committed to change unless they are actively involved in progressing and shaping it. With such active involvement in the change there are a number of potential advantages. People are more likely to accept and be enthusiastic about the change, and the organisation has the opportunity to learn from the experiences and skills of a wide range of people. The main disadvantages are that the change is likely to take longer, be more complex to manage and require more resources.

ACTIVITY 9.7

Think of a recent change in an organisation or service with which you are familiar. This can be a change that you were involved in or know about.

What was the prime purpose of the change?

What level of involvement was needed to implement this change?

Looking at the commonly used approaches described above, what approach to change best reflects the approach that was used?

Was this strategy appropriate for the type of changes sought?

Managing resistance to change

In an influential paper in the *Harvard Business Review*, Kotter and Schlesinger (1979) identified four key reasons for resistance to change:

1. parochial self-interest;

2. misunderstanding and lack of trust;

3. different assessments; and

4. low tolerance for change.

They go on to suggest some strategies for dealing with such resistance, which include:

- education and communication;

- participation and involvement;

- facilitation and support;

- negotiation and agreement;

- manipulation and co-optation; and

- implicit and explicit coercion.

Which of these strategies are chosen depends on the situation, but successful change efforts are *characterized by the skillful application of a number of these approaches often in different combinations* (Kotter and Schlesinger, 1979, p111). The skill is in assessing which approaches are most likely to be effective, given the context.

It may be useful also to think of the strategic options available to managers as existing on a continuum, from fast (on the left of the continuum) to slow (on the right of the continuum). At the fast end of the continuum are coercive, directive and expert approaches to change, while at the other end of the continuum are participative approaches to change (as illustrated in Figure 9.5).

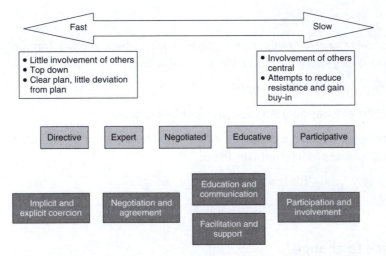

Figure 9.5 The change strategy continuum and approaches to managing change and managing resistance to change

Source: Adapted from Kotter and Schlesinger (1995) and Thurley and Wirdenius (1973)

The choice of which of these strategies to use depends on four key factors (Kotter and Schlesinger, 1979):

1. the amount and kind of resistance that is anticipated;
2. the position of the initiator in relation to the resistors;
3. the extent to which involvement is needed to achieve the change;
4. the stakes involved.

The greater the resistance that is anticipated, the more there will need to be a shift to the right of the continuum. The less power the initiator of the change has with respect to others, the greater the need to move to the left on the continuum: with greater power, a shift to the right is possible. The more that commitment from others is needed to make the change, the more there will be a need to shift to the right on the continuum. The greater the potential for risks to the organisation, the greater the need to move to the left on the continuum.

Organisational development has been influential in the change management literature, and is particularly relevant to managing complex organisational or system change (Buchanan and Huczynski, 2004; French and Bell, 1999). Van Nistelrooij and Sminia note that organisational development has *spawned a diversity of approaches and methods* (2010, p407) such as multiple stakeholder methods based on dialogue, and whole-systems approaches such as strategic scenario planning, whole-scale change and appreciative inquiry. Common to all of these approaches is the agreement that organisational development implies an attempt to understand and influence the entire organisation (or system). There is a focus on causes rather than symptoms, and participative decision-making is central to the approach. The emphasis is on the process of change, with facilitation seen as a key function (Office of the Deputy Prime Minister, 2005). In a recent publication, Van Nistelrooij and Sminia (2010, p417) propose that shared perception is one of the foremost desired outcomes of any organisational development intervention. They also argue that shared perception can be established by dialogue, and while the argument offered in this article is still at the proposition stage, the further development of organisational development as a change approach for public health professionals looks increasingly promising.

In this chapter a number of approaches to change and managing change have been discussed. However, it is inevitable that many have been omitted: for example, approaches to managing change across organisations, those that take a system-wide perspective, and emerging theories based on complexity theory. While the precise nature and shape of such approaches remains unclear (Hunter, 2003, p30), it is apparent that they would be concerned with the whole system rather than individual organisations. From this perspective, the actions of individuals and organisations are seen as interdependent and interconnected, such that *one agent's actions changes the context for other agents* (Plsek and Greenhalgh, 2001, p625). There is growing awareness that moving away from current approaches to managing change and implementing initiatives for health improvement is *an essential prerequisite* (Hunter, 2003, p30).

Chapter summary

In this chapter we began by considering why change management is important in the context of public health, health promotion and health improvement work. It was argued that public health and health promotion are essentially about achieving change at the social, environmental and political levels, as well as at an individual level, in order to improve health. Furthermore, it was noted that there has been little attention paid, within the public health and health promotion literature, to change management theory or to the development of skills to lead and manage change. Instead, attention has focused on the theoretical aspects of behaviour change and social marketing techniques. While these were viewed as legitimate areas of focus, attention was drawn to the need for public health staff to become more skilled in leading and facilitating change.

The literature on change management is vast and much of it is contradictory. There appears to be no common agreement on a framework for successful management. Debate on the nature of change and whether or not it is continuous, incremental, radical or a complex mix of these continues. Whether change is planned or emergent is another area of debate: currently, there is support for change as 'emergent', driven from the 'bottom-up'. Drivers for change include an intolerance of the wide disparities in health status and the desire to reduce inequalities in health and to maximise health gain. Other drivers for change include political imperatives, policy initiatives such as the recent decision to locate public health within local government, the desire of decision-makers for wholesale change rather than incremental evolution, an ever-changing policy context and financial imperatives such as cost pressures. Moreover, population and democratic drivers for change may act as a big influence, together with environmental considerations. The extent to which local community action at a grass roots level remains a driving force for change was questioned.

Force-field analysis, a tool that considers drivers for change, was presented as a useful tool for assessing the prospects for change. It is also useful for diagnosing and planning change interventions. Two different models of the change process, Lewin's three phases (unfreezing, changing and refreezing) and Bullock and Batten's four-phase model, focus on distinct phases of the change process. They both emphasise the need to prepare the ground, implement and then embed the change. In the English government's White Paper on public health, as well as the transition of public health from the NHS to local government and subsequent publications, the government began the process of creating the climate for change and preparing the ground for what could be viewed as radical change. More recent publications, such as details of the design of the new public health system, specifically the role and responsibilities of local government in public health, the operating model for the new executive agency Public Health England, and an overview of how the whole system will work, can be seen as the next phase of the change process.

The terms 'change strategists', 'change implementers' and 'change recipients' were introduced as distinct roles within the change process, and Kotter's eight-step model of change explained.

Stakeholder analysis and commitment planning are two tools that are widely used in managing change initiatives and projects. Different strategic approaches to change can be used, depending on the speed of change and degree of involvement required to implement the change. Kotter and Schlesinger (1979) suggest that the choice of strategies for managing resistance to change depends on four key factors: the amount and kind of resistance that is anticipated; the position of the initiator in relation to resistors; the extent to which involvement is needed to achieve the change; and the stakes involved.

Organisational development has been influential in the change management literature and is particularly relevant to managing complex organisational or system change. While there is a wide range of approaches and methods under the umbrella of organisational development, there is agreement that organisational development implies an attempt to understand and influence the entire organisation (or system).

GOING FURTHER

Office of the Deputy Prime Minister (2005) *An Organisational Development Resource Document for Local Government.* London: Office of the Deputy Prime Minister (available at **www.communities.gov.uk/documents/localgovernment/pdf/142151.pdf**; last accessed September 2011).
This document is an accessible resource produced for local government in an attempt to introduce organisational development, which was commissioned by the Office of the Deputy Prime Minister as part of the Capacity Building Programme. The aim was to produce a document that successfully unites the complex subject of organisational development with the complexity of the public sector and to present it in a way that is useful to experts and novices alike. The document was designed to meet the needs of chief executives, senior managers and senior politicians in local government and the wider public sector. The use of case study material is useful in demonstrating the practical application of organisational development change methods and processes.

Iles, V and Sutherland, K (2001) *Managing Change in the NHS: Organisational Change.* London: National Co-ordinating Centre for NHS Service Delivery and Organisation Research & Development.

Iles, V and Sutherland, K (2004) *Developing Change Management Skills.* London: National Co-ordinating Centre for NHS Service Delivery and Organisation Research & Development.
Both of these documents have been produced to provide a resource to help readers navigate some of the literature on change management and to develop their skills in managing change. The second of these publications includes a number of case studies and activities, together with a selected number of change models that may be useful.

Carnall, C (2007) *Managing Change in Organisations* (5th edn). Harlow: Prentice-Hall.
   Organised into five key parts, this book provides a comprehensive and practical explo-
   ration of change and change management in organisations. The chapters on theories
   of organisational change and change management techniques are particularly recom-
   mended for their practical relevance. The fifth part of the book has a focus on strategic
   change, and Carnall introduces a new model for organisational change, a strategic
   convergence model, which acknowledges the multiplicity of changes and the multiple
   change initiatives that take place concurrently.

References

Acheson, D (1998) *Report of the Committee of Inquiry into the Future Development of the Public Health Function*. London: HMSO.

Aldridge, H, Parekh, A, MacInnes, T and Kenway, P (2011) *Monitoring Poverty and Social Exclusion*. York: Joseph Rowntree Foundation.

Alimo-Metcalfe, B and Alban-Metcalfe, JR (2000) Heaven can wait. *Health Service Journal*, 110: 26–9.

Alvesson, M and Willmott, H (2001) *Making Sense of Management*. London: Sage.

Anderson, M (2010) *The Leadership Book*. Edinburgh: Pearson.

Antonovsky, A (1979) *Health, Stress and Coping*. San Francisco, CA: Jossey-Bass.

Armistead, C, Pettigrew, P and Aves, S (2007) Exploring leadership in multi-sectoral partnerships. *Leadership*, 3: 211–30.

Armstrong, M (2009) *Armstrong's Handbook of Human Resource Management Practice*. London: Kogan Page.

Atkinson, R (1999) Project management: cost, time and quality, two best guesses and a phenomenon. It's time to accept other success criteria. *International Journal of Project Management*, 17: 337–42.

Audit Commission (1998) *A Fruitful Partnership*. London: Audit Commission.

Audit Commission (2003) *Community Leadership: Learning from Comprehensive Performance. Assessment Briefing 1*. London: Audit Commission.

Bass, BM (1990) From transactional to transformational leadership: learning to share the vision. *Organizational Dynamics*, 18: 19–31.

Bass, BM and Avolio, B (1994) *Improving Organizational Effectiveness through Transformational Leadership*. Thousand Oaks, CA: Sage.

Bennis, W and Nanus, B (1985) *Leaders: The Strategies for Taking Charge*. London: Harper & Row.

Bentley, C (2007) *PRINCE2: A Practical Handbook* (2nd edn). Oxford: Butterworth Heinemann.

Blake, RR and Mouton, JS (1978) *The New Managerial Grid*. Houston, TX: Gulf Publishing.

Blake, RR and McCanse, AA (1991) Leadership Dilemmas: Grid Solutions. Houston, TX: Gulf Publishing.

Bolman, LG and Deal, TE (1997) *Reframing Organizations: Artistry, Choice and Leadership.* San Francisco, CA: Jossey-Bass.

Braubach, M, Jacobs, DE and Ormandy, D (eds) (2011) *Environmental Burden of Disease Associated with Inadequate Housing. A Method Guide to the Quantification of Health Effects of Selected Housing Risks in the WHO European Region.* Copenhagen: WHO Regional Office for Europe. Online at: http://www.euro.who.int/__data/assets/pdf_file/0003/142077/e95004.pdf, accessed January 2012.

Buchanan, DA and Huczynski, AA (2004) *Organizational Behaviour: An Introductory Text* (5th edn). Harlow: Pearson Education.

Bullock, RJ and Batten, D (1985) 'It's just a phase we're going through': a review and synthesis of OD phase analysis. *Group and Organization Studies,* 10: 383–412.

Burns, JM (1978) *Leadership.* New York: Harper & Row.

By, RT (2005) Organisational change management: a critical review. *Journal of Change Management,* 5: 369–80.

Cabinet Office (2010) *The Coalition: Our Programme for Government.* London: Cabinet Office.

Care Quality Commission (2011) *Dignity and Nutrition Inspection Programme: National Overview.* Newcastle Upon Tyne: Care Quality Commission. Online at: www.cqc.org.uk/sites/default/files/media/documents/20111007_dignity_and_nutrition_inspection_report.pdf, accessed 7 February 2012.

Carr, SM, Lhussier, M, Reynolds, J, Hunter, D and Hannaway, C (2009) Leadership for health improvement: implementation and evaluation. *Journal of Health, Organization and Management,* 23: 200–15.

Catford J (1997) Developing leadership for health: Our biggest blindspot. *Health Promotion International,* 12: 2–4.

Charnes, MP and Smith Tewksbury, LJ (1993) *Collaborative Management in Health Care.* San Francisco, CA: Jossey-Bass.

Chartered Institute of Personnel and Development (CIPD) (2011) *360-degree Feedback.* Online at: www.cipd.co.uk/hr-resources/factsheets/360-degree-feedback.aspx, accessed 15 November 2011.

Clark, D (1996) *Schools as Learning Communities.* London: Cassell.

Covey, S (1989) *The Seven Habits of Highly Effective People.* New York: Simon & Schuster.

Dahlgren, G and Whitehead, M (1991) *Policies and Strategies to Promote Social Equity in Health.* Stockholm: Institute of Futures Studies.

Dalrymple, J and Burke, B (2006) *Anti-oppressive Practice: Social Care and the Law*. Maidenhead: Open University Press/McGraw-Hill Education.

Deal, TE and Kennedy, A (1982) *Corporate Cultures: The Rites and Rituals of Corporate Life*. Reading, MA: Addison-Wesley.

Deal, TE and Kennedy, A (2000) *The New Corporate Cultures*. London: Texere.

Denis, JL, Lamothe, L and Langley, A (2001) The dynamics of collective leadership and strategic change in pluralistic organizations. *Academy of Management Journal*, 44: 809–37.

Department for Communities and Local Government (2008) *Practical use of the Well-Being Power*. London: Department for Communities and Local Government. Online at: www.communities.gov.uk/publications/localgovernment/localismplainenglishguide, accessed 4 February 2012.

Department of Health (2000) *The NHS Plan: A Plan for Investment, a Plan for Reform*. London: The Stationery Office.

Department of Health (2001) *Report of the Chief Medical Officer's Project to Strengthen the Public Health Function*. London: HMSO.

Department of Health (2004a) *Choosing Health: Making Healthier Choices Easier*. London: HMSO.

Department of Health (2004b) *Standards for Better Health*. London: HMSO. Online at: www.dh.gov.uk/dr_consum_dh/groups/dh_digitalassets/@dh/@en/documents/digitalasset/dh_4132991.pdf, accessed 8 February 2012.

Department of Health (2005) *Creating a Patient-led NHS: Delivering the NHS Improvement Plan*. London: HMSO.

Department of Health (2006a) *Health Challenge England: Next Steps for Choosing Health*. London: HMSO.

Department of Health (2006b) *Our Health, Our Care, Our Say: A New Direction for Community Services*. London: HMSO.

Department of Health (2008) *High Quality Care for All: NHS Next Stage Review, Final Report*. London: TSO.

Department of Health (2010a) *Equity and Excellence: Liberating the NHS*. London: HMSO.

Department of Health (2010b) *Healthy Lives, Healthy People: Our Strategy for Public Health in England*. London: HMSO.

Department of Health (2010c) *The NHS Constitution*. London: HMSO.

Online at: www.dh.gov.uk/prod_consum_dh/groups/dh_digitalassets/@dh/@en/@ps/documents/digitalasset/dh_113645.pdf, accessed 4 February 2012.

Department of Health (2011a) *Healthy Lives, Healthy People White Paper: Update and Way Forward*. London: HMSO.

Department of Health (2011b) *Healthy Lives, Healthy People: Consultation on the Funding and Commissioning Routes for Public Health*. London: HMSO.

Department of Health (2011c) *Healthy Lives, Healthy People: Transparency in Outcomes – Proposals for a Public Health Outcomes Framework*. London: HMSO.

Department of Health (2011d) Public health reform updates published, December. Online at: www.dh.gov.uk/health/2011/12/public-health-factsheets/, accessed 3 February 2012.

Department of the Environment, Transport and the Regions (1998) *Modern Local Government: In Touch with the People*. London: Department of the Environment, Transport and the Regions.

Dickinson, H, Freeman, T, Robinson, S and Williams, I (2011) Resource scarcity and priority-setting: from management to leadership in the rationing of health care? *Public Money & Management*, 31: 363–70.

Dooris, M and Hunter, D (2007), Organisations and settings for promoting public health, in Lloyd, C, Handsley S, Douglas J Earle S and Spurr S eds) *Policy and Practice in Promoting Health*. London: Sage/Open University.

Douglas, J, Jones L and Lloyd, CE (2007) The development of healthy public policy, in Lloyd, C, Handsley S, Douglas J Earle S and Spurr S (eds) *Policy and Practice in Promoting Health*. London: Sage/Open University.

Doyle, M and Smith, M (2009) Shared leadership, *Encyclopedia of Informal Education*. Online at: www.infed.org/leadership/shared_leadership.htm, accessed 2 January 2012.

Economic and Social Research Council (ESRC) Global Environmental Change Programme (2001) *Environmental Justice: Rights and Means to a Healthy Environment for All*. Special Briefing No. 7, University of Sussex.

Elbeik, S and Thomas, M (1998) *Project Skills*. Oxford: Butterworth-Heinemann.

Emmal, N and Conn, C. (2004) *Towards Community Involvement: Strategies for Health and Social Care Providers: Guide 1: Identifying the Goal and Objectives of Community Involvement*. Leeds: The Nuffield Institute for Health.

Employers Organisation (nd) *Smarter Partnerships*. Online at: www.lgpartnerships.com, accessed 10 February 2012.

Ewles, L and Simnett, I (1999) *Promoting Health: A Practical Guide*. Edinburgh: Bailliere Tindall.

Faculty of Public Health Standards Committee (2002) *Good Public Health Practice: General Professional Expectations of Public Health Professionals*. London: Faculty of Public Health.

Faculty of Public Health (2007) *Specimen job description for director of public health*. Online at: www.fph.org.uk/job_descriptions, accessed 4 February 2012.

Fiedler, FE (1967) *A Theory of Leadership Effectiveness*. New York: McGraw-Hill.

Field, M and Keller, L (1998) *Project Management*. London: Open University/ Thomson Learning.

Fisher, R, Ury, W and Patton, B (1999) *Getting to Yes: Negotiating an Agreement without Giving in* (2nd edn). London: Random House Business Books.

Frame, JD (2003) *Managing Projects in Organizations: How to Make the Best Use of Time, Techniques, and People*. San Fransisco, CA: Jossey-Bass.

Freire, P (1973) *Pedagogy of the Oppressed*. Hagerstown, MN: Harper & Row.

French, JR and Raven, B (1959) The bases of social power, in Cartwright, L and Zander, A (eds) *Group Dynamics, Research and Theory*. London: Tavistock.

French, WL and Bell, CH (1999) *Organization Development: Behavioural Science Interventions for Organization Improvement* (6th edn). Englewood Cliffs, NJ: Prentice-Hall.

Friedman, LH (2011) Changing role of public health managers and leaders, in Burke, RE and Friedman, LH, *Essentials of Management and Leadership in Public Health*. Sudbury, MA: Jones and Bartlett Learning.

Fulop, L, Linstead, S and Dunford, R (2004) Leading and managing, in Linstead, S, Fulop, L and Lilley, S (eds) *Management and Organization: A Critical Text*. Basingstoke: Palgrave Macmillan.

Gardner, JW (1990) *On Leadership*. New York: The Free Press.

Geddes, M (1998) *Achieving Best Value through Partnership*, Best Value Series No. 7. Coventry and London: University of Warwick/Department of the Environment, Transport and the Regions.

General Medical Council (GMC) (2006) *Good Medical Practice*. London: GMC.

Gibson, C (1991) A concept analysis of empowerment. *Journal of Advanced Nursing*, 16: 354–61.

Goleman, D (1998) *Working with Emotional Intelligence*. New York: Bantham Books.

Goleman, D (2000) Leadership that gets results. *Harvard Business Review*, 78: 78–90.

Goleman, D, Boyatzis, R and McKee, A (2001) Primal leadership: the hidden driver of great performance. *Harvard Business Review*, 79: 42–51.

Goleman, D, Boyatzis, R and McKee, A (2002) *Primal Leadership: Realizing the Power of Emotional Intelligence*. Boston, MA: Harvard Business School Press.

Goleman, D, Boyatzis, R and McKee, A (2003) *The New Leaders*. London: Time Warner Paperbacks.

Graham, H and Kelly, M (2004) *Health Inequalities: Concepts, Frameworks and Policy*. London: Health Development Agency.

Green, J and Tones, K (2010) *Health Promotion: Planning and Strategies* (2nd edn). London: Sage.

Grint, K (1997) *Leadership: Classical, Contemporary and Critical Approaches.* Oxford: Oxford University Press.

Gronn, P (2002) Distributed leadership, in Leithwood, K, Hallinger, P, Seashore-Louis, K, Furmann-Brown, G, Gronn, P, Mulford, W and Riley, K (eds) *Second International Handbook of Educational Leadership and Administration.* Dordrecht: Kluwer.

Grundy, T (1993) *Managing Strategic Change.* London: Kogan Page.

Handsley, S (2007) The potential for promoting public health at a local level: community strategies and health improvement, in Lloyd, C, Handsley, S, Douglas, J, Earle, S and Spurr, S (eds) *Policy and Practice in Promoting Health.* London: Sage.

Handy, CB (1988) *Understanding Voluntary Organisations.* London: Penguin.

Handy, CB (1993) *Understanding Organizations* (4th edn). London: Penguin.

Handy, C (1999[1976]) *Understanding Organisations.* Harmondsworth: Penguin.

Hannaway, C, Plsek, P and Hunter, DJ (2007) Developing Leadership and Management for Health, in Hunter, DJ (ed.) *Managing for Health.* London: Routledge.

Hartley, J with Lawton, A (1998) *Leading Communities: Competencies for Effective Community Leadership.* Luton: Local Government Management Board.

Hartley, J, Martin, J and Benington, J (2008) *A Review of the Literature for Health Care Professionals, Managers and Researchers.* Warwick: Institute of Governance and Public Management, Warwick Business School, University of Warwick.

Heifetz, RA (1994) *Leadership without Easy Answers.* Cambridge, MA: Harvard University Press.

Heifetz, RA and Laurie, DL? (1997) The work of leadership. *Harvard Business Review*, 75: 124–34.

Hersey, P and Blanchard, KH (1988[1969]) *Management of Organizational Behavior: Utilizing Human Resources* (5th edn). Englewood Cliffs, NJ: Prentice-Hall.

Hodgkinson, GP and Sparrow, PR (2002) *The Competent Organisation: A Psychological Analysis of the Strategic Management Process.* Buckingham: Open University Press.

Homan, M (2008) *Promoting Community Change: Making it Happen in the Real World* (4th edn). Belmont, CA: Thompson Learning.

Hosking, DM (1997) Organizing, leadership and skilful process, in Grint, K (ed.) *Leadership: Classical, Contemporary and Critical Approaches.* Oxford: Oxford University Press.

Hudson, M. (1999) *Managing Without Profit.* Harmondsworth: Penguin.

Hunter, DJ (2003) Public health policy, in Orme, J, Powell J, Taylor, P, Harrison, H and Grey, M (eds) *Public Health for the 21st Century: New Perspectives on Policy, Participation and Practice*. Maidenhead: McGraw-Hill Education/Open University Press.

Hunter, DJ (ed.) (2007) *Managing for Health*. Abingdon: Routledge.

Iles, V and Sutherland, K (2001) *Managing Change in the NHS: Organisational Change*. London: National Coordinating Centre for NHS Service Delivery and Organisation Research & Development.

Improvement and Development Agency (IDeA) (2009) *Setting the Standard for Partnerships*. Online at: www.idea.gov.uk/idk/alo/21134954, accessed March 2012.

Improvement and Development Agency (IDeA) (2010) *A Glass Half-full: How an Asset Approach Can Improve Community Health and Well-being*. London: IDeA.

Kanter, RM, Stein, BA and Jick, TD (1992) *The Challenge of Organizational Change: How Companies Experience It and Leaders Guide It*. New York: Free Press.

Kemp, L, Fordham, R, Robson, A, Bate, A, Donaldson, C, Baughan, S, Ferguson, B and Brambleby, P (2008) *Road Testing Programme Budgeting and Marginal Analysis (PBMA) in three English Regions: Hull (Diabetes), Newcastle (CAHMS), Norfolk (Mental Health)*. York: York & Humber Public Health Observatory. Online at: www.yhpho.org.uk/resource/item.aspx?RID=10049, accessed September 2011.

Kirkpatrick, SA and Locke, E A (1991) Leadership: do traits matter? *Academy of Management Executive*, 5: 48–59.

Kotter, J (1995) Leading change: why transformation efforts fail. *Harvard Business Review*, 73: 59–67.

Kotter, J (1996) *Leading Change*. Boston, MA: Harvard Business School Press.

Kotter, JP (1990) *A Force for Change: How Leadership Differs from Management*. New York: Free Press.

Kotter, JP and Schlesinger, LA (1979) Choosing strategies for change. *Harvard Business Review*, 57: 106–14.

Kouzes, J and Posner, B (1987) *The Leadership Challenge: How to Get Extraordinary Things Done in Organizations*. San Francisco, CA: Jossey-Bass.

Kouzes, JM and Posner, BZ (1995) *The Leadership Challenge* (3rd edn). San Francisco, CA: Jossey-Bass.

Kouzes, J and Posner, B (2007) *The Leadership Challenge* (4th edn). San Francisco, CA: Jossey-Bass.

Kretzmann, J and McKnight, J (1997) *Building Communities from the Inside Out: A Path Toward Finding and Mobilizing Community Assets*. Evanston, IL: Asset-Based Community Development Institute.

Labonte, R (1998) *A Community Development Approach to Health Promotion: A Background Paper on Practice Tensions, Strategic Models and Accountability Requirements for Health Authority Work in the Broad Determinants of Health.* Prepared for Health Education Board of Scotland, Research Unit on Health and Behaviour Change. Edinburgh: University of Edinburgh.

Lavarack, G (2004) *Health Promotion Practice: Power and Empowerment.* London: Sage.

Lawrence, PR and Lorsch, JW (1967) *Organizations and Environment.* Cambridge, MA: Harvard University Press.

Leach, S and Wilson, D (2000) *Local Political Leadership.* Bristol: Policy Press.

Ledwith, M (2005) *Community Development: A Critical Approach.* Bristol: Policy Press.

Ledwith, M (2007) Reclaiming the radical agenda: a critical approach to community development. *Concept* 17: 8–12. Online at: www.infed.org/community/critical_community_development.htm, accessed September 2011.

Lewin, K (1951) *Field Theory in Social Science.* London: Harper & Row.

Lewin, K, Lippitt, R and White, RK (1939) Patterns of aggressive behaviour in experimentally created social climates, *Journal of Social Psychology*, 1939, 10: 271–299.

Linstead, S, Fulop, L and Lilley, S (eds) (2004) *Management and Organization: A Critical Text.* Basingstoke: Palgrave Macmillan.

Longest, BB (2004) *Managing Health Programs and Projects.* San Francisco, CA: John Wiley & Sons/Jossey-Bass.

Lowndes, V (2004) Reformers or recidivists? Has local government really changed?, in Stoker, G and Wilson, D (eds) *British Local Government into the 21st Century.* Basingstoke: Palgrave.

Luke, LS (1997) *Catalytic Leadership: Strategies for an Interconnected World.* San Francisco, CA: Jossey-Bass.

McKimm, J and Philips, K (2009) *Leadership and Management in Integrated Services.* Exeter: Learning Matters.

McNaught, A (2009) Leadership in community health development, in Stewart, J and Cornish, Y (eds) *Professional Practice in Public Health.* Exeter: Reflect Press.

Madden, A (2010a) The community leadership and place-shaping roles of English local government: synergy or tension? *Public Policy and Administration*, 25:175–93.

Madden, A (2010b) Making sense of community leadership: a case study of local leadership, community empowerment and the enrichment of the public realm. *PSA Conference Proceedings.* Online at: www.psa.ac.uk/journals/pdf/5/2010/551_617.pdf, accessed September 2011.

Markwell, S, Watson, J, Speller, V, Platt, S and Younger, T (2003) *The Working Partnership Book 1: Introduction*. London: Health Development Agency.

Marmot, M (2007) Achieving health equity: from root causes to fair outcomes. *The Lancet*, 370: 1153–63.

Marmot, M (2010) *Fair Society, Healthy Lives: The Marmot Review*. London: The Marmot Review.

Martin, V (2001) *Managing in Health and Social Care*. London: Routledge.

Martin, V (2002) *Managing Projects in Health and Social Care.* Abingdon: Routledge.

Martin, V (2003) *Leading Change in Health and Social Care*. London: Routledge.

Martin, V, Charlesworth, J and Henderson, ES (2010) *Managing in Health and Social Care* (2nd edn). Abingdon: Routledge.

Maylor, H (2005) *Project Management* (3rd edn). Harlow: Pearson Education.

Mento, AJ, Jones RM and Dirndorfer, W (2002) A change management process: Grounded in both theory and practice. *Journal of Change Management*, 3: 45–59.

Mintzberg, H (1971) Managerial work: analysis from observation. *Management Science*, 18: 97–110.

Mintzberg, H (1973) *The Nature of Managerial Work.* New York: Harper & Row.

Mintzberg, H (1979) *The Structuring of Organizations*: *A synthesis of the Research*. Englewood Cliffs, NJ: Prentice-Hall.

Mintzberg, H (1983a) *Power in and Around Organisations*. Englewood Cliffs, NJ: Prentice-Hall.

Mintzberg, H (1983b) *Structures in Fives: Designing Effective Organisations.* Englewood Cliffs. NJ: Prentice-Hall.

Mullins, LJ (2002) *Management and Organisational Behaviour* (6th edn). Harlow: Pearson Education.

Naidoo, J and Wills, J (2009) *Foundations for Health Promotion*. London: Balliere Tindall Elsevier.

National Occupational Standards (2009) *National Occupational Standards for Community Development.* London: Lifelong Learning UK.

Nelson, L (2003) A case study in organizational change: implications for theory. *The Learning Organization*, 10: 18–30.

National Institute for Clinical Excellence (NICE) (2007) *Behaviour Change (PH6)*. London: NICE.

Northouse, PG (1997) *Leadership: Theory and Practice.* Thousand Oaks, CA: Sage.

Northouse, PG (2001) *Leadership, Theory and Practice* (2nd edn). Thousand Oaks, CA: Sage.

Nutbeam, D and Wise, M (2002) Structures and strategies for public health intervention, in Detels, R, McEwan, J, Beaglehole, R and Tanaka, H (eds) *Oxford Textbook of Public Health*, Vol. 3 (4th edn). Oxford: Oxford University Press.

Office of the Deputy Prime Minister (2005) *An Organisational Development Resource Document for Local Government*. London: Office of the Deputy Prime Minister. Online at: www.communities.gov.uk/documents/localgovernment/pdf/142151.pdf, accessed September 2011.

Pendleton, D and King, J (2002) Values and leadership. *British Medical Journal* 325: 1352–5.

Pettigrew, A and Whipp, R (1993) Understanding the environment, in Mabey, C and Mayon-White, B (eds) *Managing Change* (2nd edn). London: Paul Chapman Publishing.

Plant, R (1978) Community: concept, conception and ideology. *Politics and Society*, 8: 79–107.

Plsek, PE and Greenhalgh, T (2001) The challenge of complexity in health care. *British Medical Journal*, 323: 625–8.

Popay, J (2010) Community empowerment and health improvement, in Morgan, A, Davies, M and Ziglio, E (eds) *Health Assets in a Global Context: Theory Methods Action*. New York: Springer.

Pratt, J, Plamping, D and Gordon, P (1998) *Partnership: Fit for Purpose?* London: The King's Fund.

PRINCE2 (nd) Online at: http://webarchive.nationalarchives.gov.uk/20110822131357/http://www.ogc.gov.uk/methods_prince_2.asp, accessed 4 February 2012.

Pugh, DS (1988) *The convergence of international organisational behaviour*. Invited paper to the British Psychological Society Conference, London, and Open University School of Management Working Paper No. 2/90.

Rao, M (2006) Developing public health leadership. *Ph.com: Newsletter of the Faculty of Public Health*, June. Online at: www.fph.org.uk/uploads/phcom_june06.pdf, accessed 23 October 2011.

Rychetnik, L, Frommer, M, Hawe, P and Shiell, A (2002) Criteria for evaluating evidence on public health interventions. *Journal of Epidemiology and Community Health*, 56: 119–27.

Rychetnik, L, Hawe, P, Waters, E, Barratt, A and Frommer, M (2004) A glossary for evidence based public health. *Journal of Epidemiology and Community Health*, 58: 538–45.

Sacker, A, Firth, D, Fitzpatrick, R, Lynch, K and Bartley, M (2000) Comparing health inequality in men and women: Prospective study of mortality 1986–96. *British Medical Journal*, 320: 1303–7.

Senior, B (2002) *Organisational Change* (2nd edn) Harlow: Pearson Education.

Shannon CE and Weaver W (1949) *A Mathematical Model of Communication.* Urbana, IL: University of Illinois Press.

Shaw, M (2008) Community development and the politics of community. *Community Development Journal*, 43: 24–36.

Sisson, K and Storey, J (2000) *The Realities of Human Resource Management.* Buckingham: Open University Press.

Smith, K, Bambra, C, Perkins, N, Hunter, D, Joyce, K and Blenkinsopp, E (2008) *Partnerships in Public Health: A Healthy Outcome? Summary Findings of a Systematic Literature Review.* Durham: Durham University School of Medicine and Health. Online at: www.dur.ac.uk/resources/public.health/news/PartnershipWorkingin-PublicHealth-SummaryLiteratureReviewFindings.pdf, accessed July 2011.

Smith, MK (2006) Community development. Online at: www.infed.org/community/b-comdv.htm, accessed September 2011.

Spillane, JP (2005) Distributed leadership. *The Educational Forum*, 69: 143–50.

Stewart, M (2002) *Systems Governance: Towards Effective Partnership Working.* Paper to the Health Development Agency Seminar Series on Tackling Health Inequalities. Bristol: The Cities Research Centre, University of the West of England. Online at: www.hda.nhs.uk/evidence, accessed November 2011.

Sullivan, H (2008) *Meta Evaluation of the Local Government Modernisation Agenda.* London: Department of Communities and Local Government.

Sullivan, H, Downe, J, Entwistle, T and Sweeting, D (2006) The three challenges of community leadership. *Local Government Studies*, 32: 489–508.

Tannenbaum, R and Schmidt, W (1958) How to choose a leadership pattern. *Harvard Business Review*, 36: 95–101.

Tannenbaum, R and Schmidt, W (1973) How to choose a leadership pattern. *Harvard Business Review*, 51: 162–80.

Taylor, M (2003) *Public Policy in the Community.* Basingstoke: Palgrave.

The King's Fund and Rowling, E (eds) (2011) *The Future of Leadership and Management in the NHS: No More Heroes.* London: The King's Fund Commission on Leadership and Management.

Thomas, D (1983) *The Making of Community Work.* London: George Allen.

Thurley, K and Wirdenius, H (1973) *Supervision: A Reappraisal.* London: Heinemann.

Tichy, NM and Ulrich, DO (1984) The leadership challenge: a call for the transformational leader. *Sloan Management Review*, 26: 59–68.

Trice, HM and Beyer, JM (1984) Studying organizational cultures through rites and rituals. *Academy of Management Review*, 9: 653–69.

Turnbull James, K (2011) *Leadership in Context: Lessons from New Leadership Theory and Current Leadership Development Practice.* Online at: www.kingsfund. org.uk/publications/articles/leadership_papers/leadership_theory.html, accessed November 2011.

Twelvetrees, A (1991) *Community Work.* Basingstoke: Palgrave Macmillan.

Van Maurik, J (2001) *Writers on Leadership.* London: Penguin.

Van Nistelrooij, A and Sminia, H (2010) Organization development: What's actually happening? *Journal of Change Management*, 10: 407–20.

Wanless, D (2002) *Securing Our Future Health: Taking a Long-term View.* London: HM Treasury.

Wanless, D (2004) *Securing Good Health for the Whole Population: Final Report.* London: HM Treasury.

Weber, M (1947) *The Theory of Social and Economic Organization.* New York: Oxford University Press.

Wenger, E and Snyder, W (2000) Communities of practice: the organizational frontier. *Harvard Business Review*, 78: 139–45.

Wills, J (2009) Community development in public health and primary care, in Sines, D, Saunders, M and Forbes-Burford, J (eds) *Community Health Care Nursing* (4th edn). Chichester: Wiley-Blackwell.

Winslow, C (1920) The untilled fields of public health. *Science*, 51: 23–33.

World Health Organization (WHO) (1984) *Health Promotion: Concepts and Principles.* Copenhagen: WHO Regional Office for Europe. Online at: http://whqlibdoc.who.int/euro/-1993/ICP_HSR_602__m01.pdf, accessed 12 December 2011.

World Health Organization (WHO) (1988) Second International Conference on Health Promotion, Adelaide, South Australia, 5–9 April.

World Health Organization (WHO) (2008) *Commission on Social Determinants of Health.* Geneva: WHO.

Zaleznik A (1977) Managers and leaders: are they different? *Harvard Business Review*, 55: 67–78.

Index